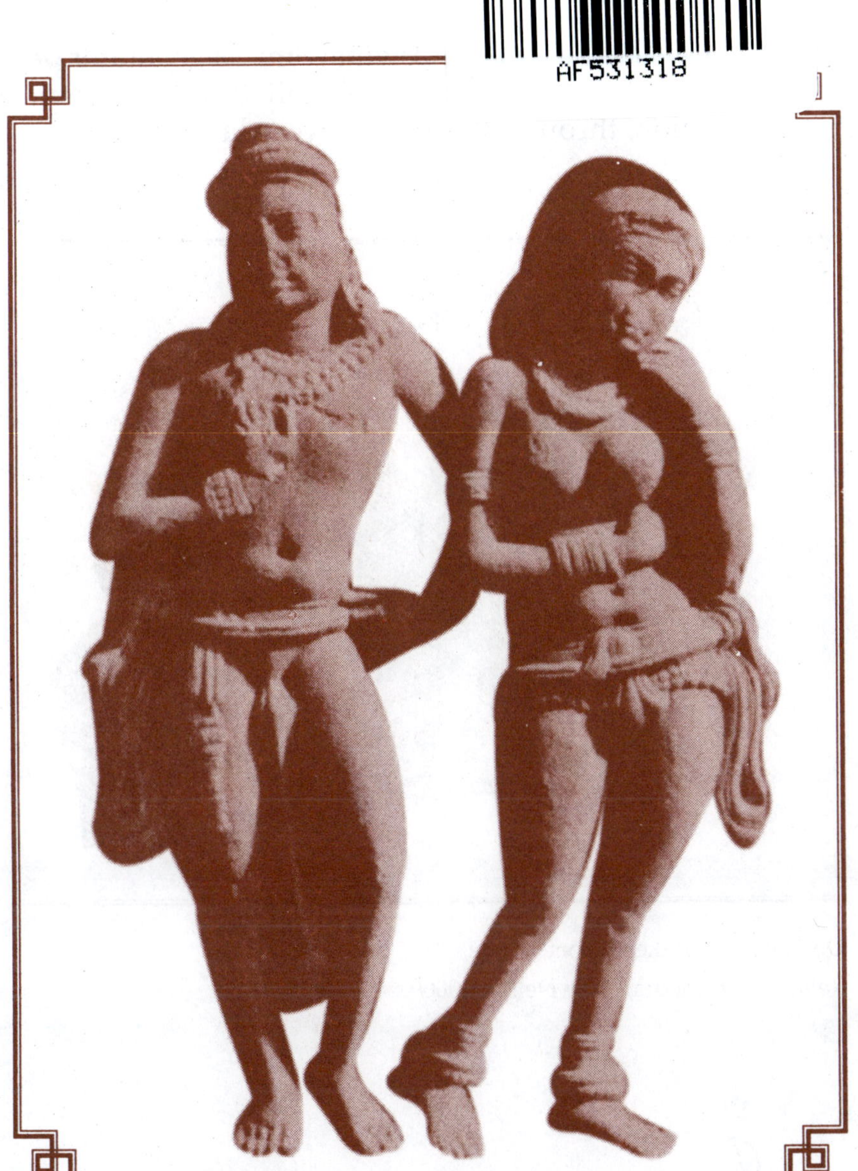

INDIA BOOKVARSITY

LOTUS CHOICES

Editor: Mahendra Kulasrestha

In India Eros is not the Original Sin; as generator of life, it holds supreme and pervades all its aspects from religion, through the arts, to everyday ethics.

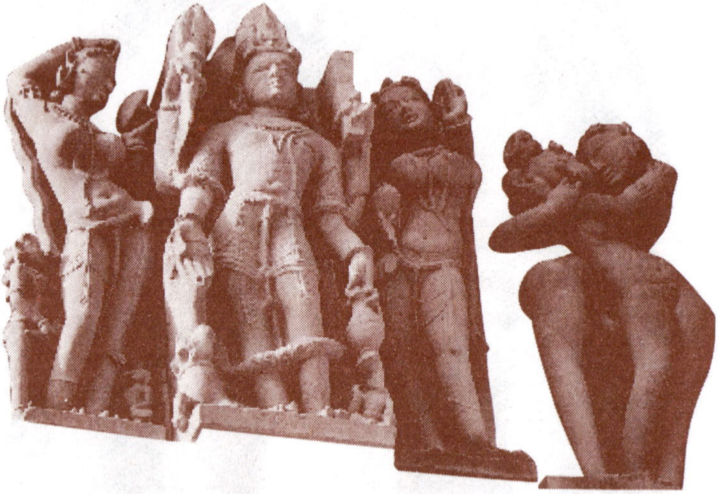

Designed by Rakesh Goel
Reliable Infomedia, New Delhi-110009.

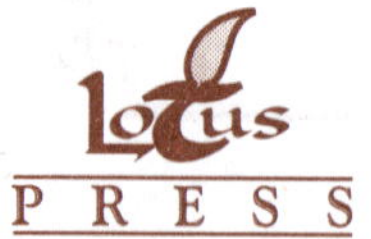

4263/3, Ansari Road, Darya Ganj
New Delhi-110002

VATSYAYANA'S KAMASUTRA SELECT

AND HIS TIMES

A cultured person's handbook of good and gracious life

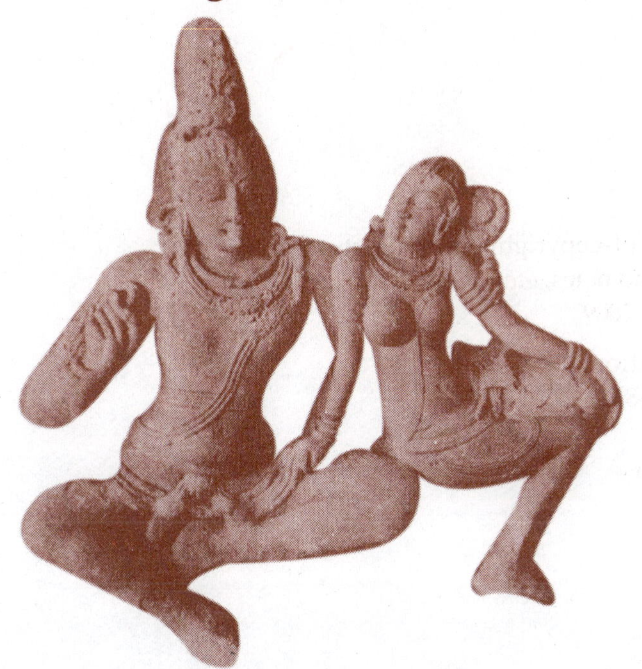

Translation in English by
SIR RICHARD BURTON
and F. F. ARBUTHNOT
and
the study of his times by
PROF. H. C. CHAKLADAR

Sources:

1. Sir Richard Burton and F. F. Arbuthnot's translation in English, published by the Kama Shastra Society, London and Varanasi, 1883.

and

2. Prof. H. C. Chakladar's *Sidelights of Social Life in Ancient India: Studies in Vatsyayana's Kamasutra,* published by Greater India Society, Calcutta, 1929.

❖❖

First Edition 2009
ISBN: 81-8382-173-1

❖❖

Published by: Lotus Press, New Delhi-110002
Lasertypeset by: Reliable Infomedia, New Delhi-110009
Printed in India by: Saras Graphics, Delhi

'The Kamasutra, attributed to the sage Vatsyayana and written in the early centuries of the Christian era...(is a) remarkable work (which) gives...detailed instruction on erotic technique and much very valuable information about the life of the ancient Indian.'

'Sexuality was not looked on as a mere vent for the animal passions of the male, but as a refined mutual relationship. There was much tenderness in love-making. Vatsyayana gives a detailed example of the courtship of a newly married bride for her husband, which would win the approval of most modern psychologists.'

– A. L. Basham

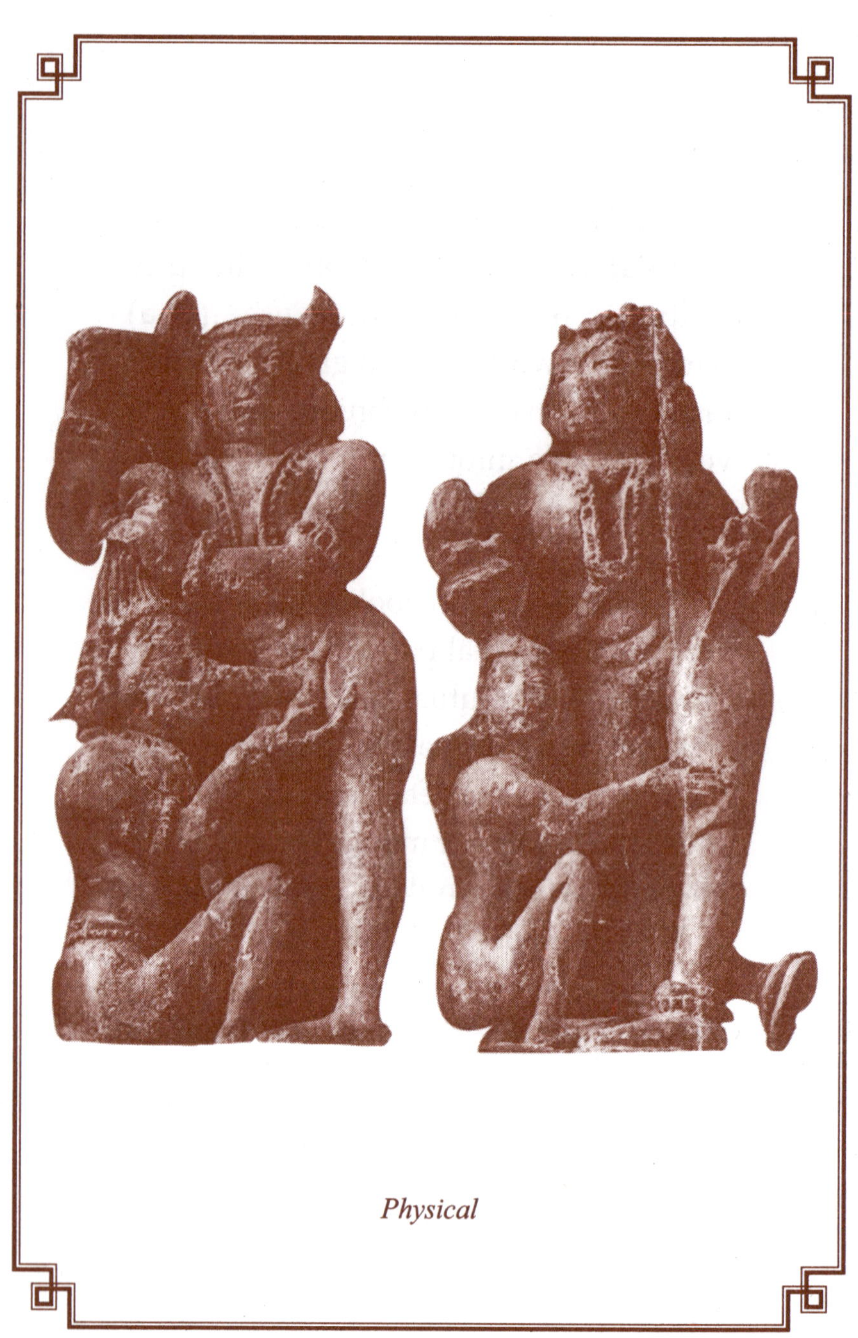

Physical

Editorspeak

A Balanced View

Kamasutra and Khajuraho - none of the likes of these exist anywhere else in the world. No wonder that when in the nineteenth century, Richard Burton, a middle-level soldier of the East India Company establishment in India of those times, discovered fragments of the treatise, he was overwhelmed by excitement and left no stone unturned, as the legend goes, to not only acquire the complete text, but translated it into his community/race's language for their use and benefit. The credit for popularising the work all over the then known world goes entirely and absolutely to him, and to him only, later on known as 'Sir' Richard Burton, with the knighthood awarded to the soldier for this as well as perhaps for other work in the company's service. Hurrah to him! even after so many years.

Dear Sir Richard Burton of the Kamasutra in English fame or notoriety in real life looked like a monster, a satan out to demonise the world, 'cruel, treacherous, with eyes like a wild beast's' in the words of the poet Wilfrid Blunt, but with an unusually restless intellect, who after being rusticated from the Oxford University, wandered long, finally reaching Baroda in far away India in 1842, and joined the Bombay Native Infantry under the command of the famous Sir Charles Napier. He fought little, but roamed in the dark lanes of Karachi fraternising with their inhabitants, female as well as male, other service-providers in various imaginable ways to the forces and keeping his own favourites at his bungalow itself, which his colleagues did not much appreciate. But Napier, recognising his special talents, used him as a spy which further helped him in developing his talents in academic erotology. He prepared confidential reports for the army on the soldiers', activities in the area, bringing out the startling fact that many of the brothels catered exclusively to the needs of the homos. He himself in the process caught some of the diseases, fell seriously ill and left for England in 1849.

He had now discovered his life's mission, and since 'mind over matter' is an eternal truth, he wandered and lived for another forty years, researching and writing, with his assistant Foster Arbuthnot the Kamasutra of Vatsyayana as well as the 'Anang-Rang' of Kalyanamalla and 'The Perfumed Garden' – which may be called the Arabian or Muslim Kamasutra of Sheikh Nefzawi. He for this purpose, founded the Kama Shastra Society, with offices in London and Banaras, and printers in Paris, Amsterdam and London. The venture drew attention, but the books took several decades to be popular owing to the prevailing Victorian mores of social behaviour. It may be noted that his wife Isabel did not approve of his work and destroyed large parts of the mss or corrected them according to her thinking before sending them to press – otherwise, it is quite possible that not only the volume of the work but its spice-element would also have been more. It is interesting that the day Richard Burton completed the very important new section of 'The Perfumed Garden', and gave it his finishing touches, he passed away. This time also Isabel consigned the pages to fire.

•

The Kamasutra is one book which everyone wants to read, but not in the open. It therefore has an immense market all over the world, a great money-spinner in the field of books. Most publishers for this reason, including my own, wanted to do an edition, and those who have done it, have embellished it with colour pics of the positions, which then become more important than the text itself, and are purchased chiefly to look at them when there is no one around.

In course of time the word 'Kamasutra' became a brand and started being used for a variety of purposes. The present editor has always felt that the work should be presented in the correct perspective, supported chiefly by the erotic sculptures and other art works widely available in our gorgeous temples all over the country. It is noteworthy that religious themes, including the gods and goddesses, are sufficiently provocative, a special feature of Indian art-culture. The beautiful drawings of the Buddhist caves of Ajanta, the statue of Lord Mahavira at Sravanabelagola etc. are cases in point. The Surasundaries around the upper structures of Konarak are beauty personified. The explicit action sculptures of Khajuraho, some of the Konarak itself and similar others form a category of their own, an expression of the widest or wildest possibilities of human life and culture.

Therefore I looked out for some research material related to Vatsyayana, which would throw light on other aspects of life in Indian society. I did, fortunately, find a work by Prof. Haran Chandra Chakladar of the ancient Indian history department of Calcutta University, published under the auspices of the Greater India Society run by the famous Dr. Kalidas Nag. Prof. Chakladar's study is remarkable in the respect that it undertakes a subject the like of which is generally ignored by research scholars. He seems to have a penchant for such subjects because the other study he has published is related to the occupation of Aryans in Eastern India, another interesting but ignored subject in the development of the country's culture.

I decided to introduce Vatsyayana's Kamasutra with select portions of this significant work and prepare the reader before going through the main work. It not only puts the whole in perspective, but, taken independently, provides interesting information on the social structure in Indian towns in the first centuries of the Christian era. One finds it heartening to learn that India was very prosperous in those times and the city-bred persons were men of 'considerable intellectual culture and aesthetic refinement.....wealth and riches were flowing into India through an extensive commerce with the east and the west.'

But the pattern of life described in the Kamasutra was not spread all over the country, the general ideals of the society were the same as propounded in the Dharmashastras, and in fact, the Eros aspect was an integral part of it; the Kamasutra itself elaborates it in so many words. Eros has never been regarded as a sin - or Original Sin as in Judaic-Christianity, which has resulted in the special problems of the modern West-influenced world-society. India's is a basically different concept which should be properly comprehended to appreciate these and related matters.

The case of the Ganikas - normally taken as common prostitutes - should be underlined to make it clear. They were educated and cultured, with special proficiency in various arts, which were as many as 64 in number, and were really and truly respected. Amrapali was one such whom even the Buddha did not hesitate to accept as a disciple. In comparision to other known cultures in the world, our values and behaviour were more natural and balanced, and very liberal especially in regard to women. It would seem that the situation has not much changed despite the passage of two millennia. Our only black spot has been and is the untouchability aspect of the caste system.

This book is not intended to provide titillation to one's senses in his spare time, but to give him a realistic, matter of fact knowledge of the subject, as given by Vatsyayana in his brief aphoristic style, which is very prosaic and just indicative of the details. Had the learned Yashodhara not elaborated it in his famous 'Jayamangala' commentary, it would have been lost in the sands of time

We have also included selections from the original Sanskrit of the Kamasutra to give a correct idea of the work to the reader at the insistence of our artist Rakesh Goel, who has also composed the work at Reliable Infomedia. He has worked hard at the project, and especially at giving it a sober yet attractive look.

CONTENTS

1.

The Kamasutra in Sanskrit

2.

The Kamasutra in English

3.

Indian Life in the Times of Vatsyayana

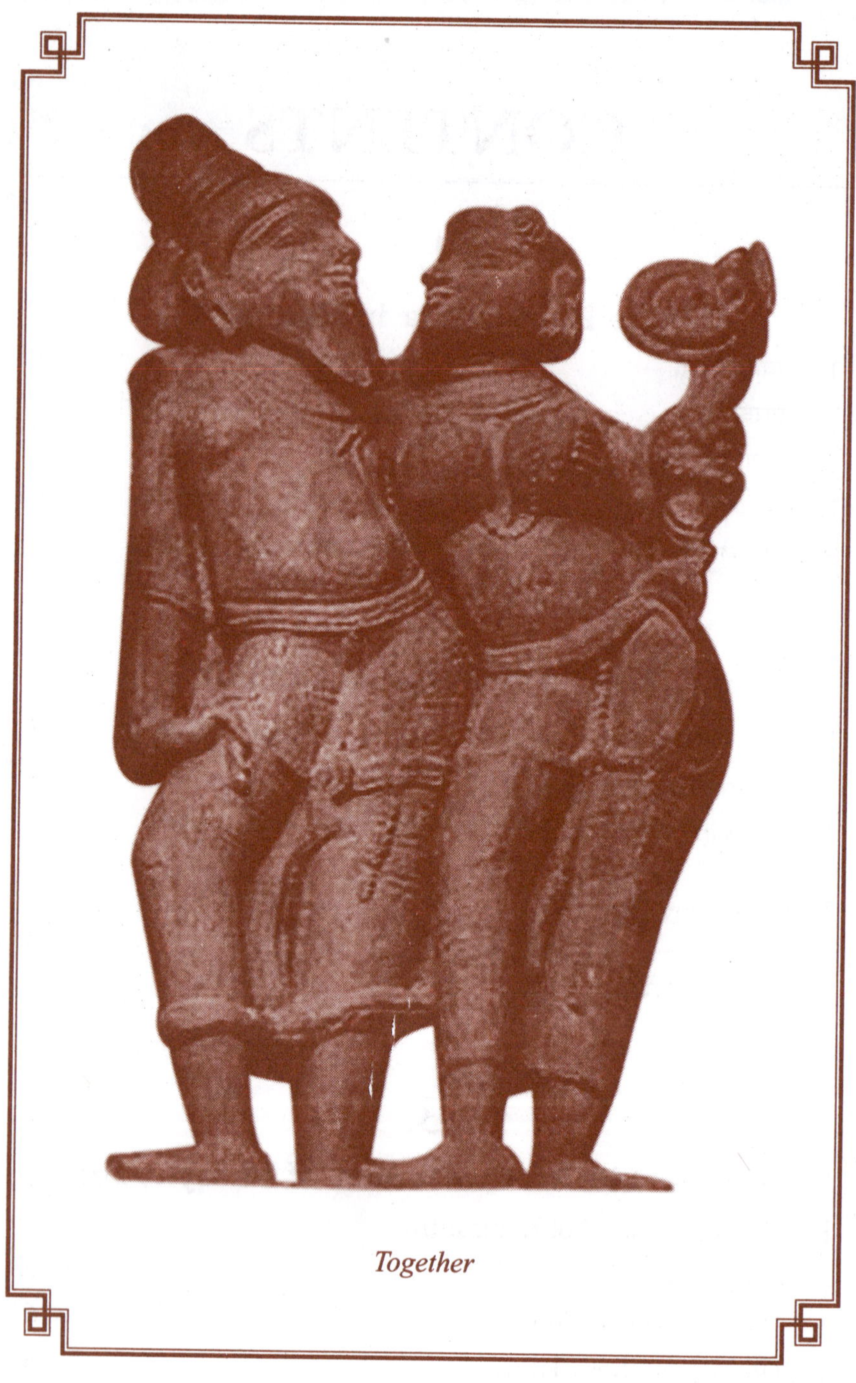

Together

1

The Kamasutra of Vatsyayana

Original in Sanskrit Abridged

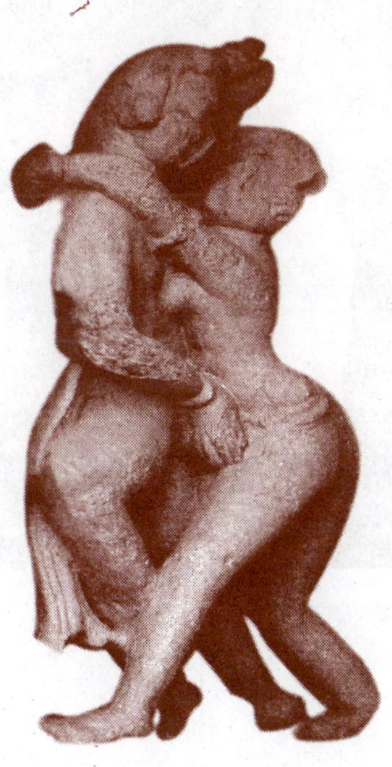

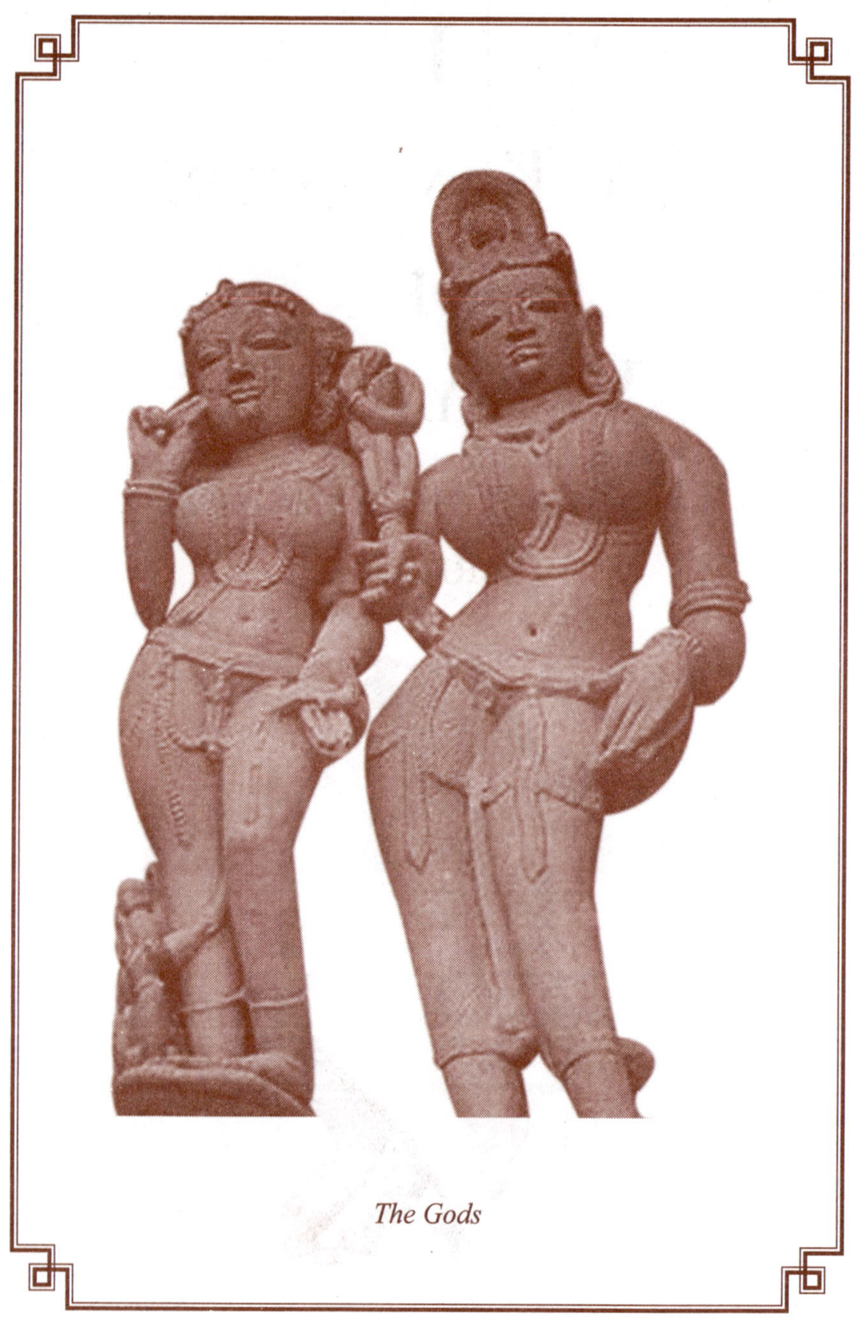

The Gods

त्रिवर्गप्रतिपत्ति

शतायुर्वै पुरुषो विभज्य कालमन्योन्यानुबद्धं
परस्परस्यानुपघातकं त्रिवर्ग सेवेत ।।

बाल्ये विद्याग्रहणादीनर्थान् ।
कामं च यौवने।
स्थाविरे धर्म मोक्षं च ।

अनित्यत्वादायुषो यथोपपादं वा सेवेत् ।
ब्रह्मचर्यमेव त्वा विद्याग्रहणात् ।

अलौकिकत्वाद्दृष्टार्थत्वादप्रवृत्तानां
यज्ञादीनां शास्त्रात्प्रवर्तनम्,
लौकित्वाद्दृष्टार्थत्वाच्च प्रवृत्तेभ्यश्च मांसभक्षणादिभ्यः
शास्त्रादेव निवारणं धर्मः ।

विद्याभूमिहिरण्यपशुधान्यभाण्डोपस्करमित्रादी ।
नामर्जनमर्जितस्य विवर्धनमर्थः ।

श्रोत्रत्वक्चक्षुर्जिह्वाघ्राणानामात्मसंयुक्तेन मनसाधिष्ठितानां स्वेषु स्वेषु विषयेष्वानुकूल्यतः प्रवृत्तिः कामः।

स्पर्शविशेषविषयात्वस्याभिमानिकसुखानुविद्धा फलवत्यर्थप्रतीतिः प्राधान्यात्कामः।
तं कामसूत्रागन्नरिकजनसमवायाच्च प्रतिपद्येत।
एषां समवाये पूर्वः पूर्वो गरीयान् ।

तिर्यग्योनिष्वपि तु स्वयं प्रवृत्तत्वात् कामस्य नित्यत्वाच्च न शास्त्रेण कृत्यमस्तीत्याचार्याः ।

संप्रयोगपराधीनत्वात् स्त्रीपुंसयोरुपायमपेक्षते ।
सा चोपायप्रतिपत्तिः कामसूत्रादिति वात्स्यायनः ।

शरीरस्थितिहेतुत्वादाहारसधर्माणो हि कामाः फलभूताश्च धर्मार्थयोः ।

बोद्धव्यं तु दोषेष्विव। नहि भिक्षुकाः ।
सन्तीति स्थाल्यो नाधिश्रीयन्ते।

एवमर्थं च कामं च धर्मं चोपाचरन्नारः।
इहामुत्र च निःशल्यमत्यन्तं सुखमश्नुते ॥

विद्यासमुद्देश

अभ्यासप्रयोज्यांश्च चातुःषष्टिकान् योगान्
कन्या रहस्येकाकिन्यभ्यसेत् ।

गीतम्, वाद्यम्, नृत्यम्, आलेख्यम्, विशेषकच्छेद्यम्, तण्डुलकुसुमवलिविकाराः, पुष्पास्तरणम्, दशनवसनाङ्गरागः, मणिभूमिकाकर्म, शयनरचनम्, उदकवाद्यम्, उदकाघातः, चित्राश्च योगाः, माल्यग्रथनविकल्पाः, शेखरकापीडयोजनम्, नेपथ्यप्रयोगाः, कर्णपत्रभङ्गाः, गन्धयुक्तिः, भूषणयोजनम्, ऐन्द्रजालाः, कौचुमाराश्च योगाः, हस्तलाघवम्, विचित्र-शाकयूषभक्ष्यविकारक्रिया, पानकरसरागासवयोजनम्, सूची-वानकर्माणि, सूत्रक्रीडा, वीणाडमरुकवाद्यानि, प्रहेलिका, प्रतिमाला, दुर्वाचकयोगाः, पुस्तकवाचनम्, नाटकाख्यायि-कादर्शनम्, काव्यसमस्यापूरणम्, पट्टिकावावेत्रविकल्पाः, तक्षकर्माणि, तक्षणम्, वास्तुविद्या, रूप्यपरीक्षा, धातु-वादः, मणिरागाकरज्ञानम्, वृक्षायुर्वेदयोगाः, मेषकुक्कुटलावक-युद्धविधिः, शुकसारिकाप्रलापनम्, उत्सादने संवाहने केश-मर्दने च कौशलम्, अक्षरमुष्टिकाकथनम् । म्लेच्छितविकल्पाः, देशभाषाविज्ञानम्, पुष्पशकटिका, निमितज्ञानम् यन्त्र-मातृका, धारणमातृका, सम्पाठ्यम्, मानसी काव्यक्रिया,

अभिधानकोशः, छन्दोज्ञानम्, क्रियाकल्पः, छलितकयोगाः, वस्त्रगोपनानि, द्यूतविशेषः, आकर्षक्रीडा, बालक्रीडनकानि, वैनयिकीनाम्, वैजयिकीनाम् व्यायामिकीनां च विद्यानां ज्ञानम्, इति चतुःषष्टिरङ्ग.विद्याः । कामसूत्रस्यावयविन्यः ।

आभिरभ्युच्छ्रिता वेश्या शीलरूपगुणान्विता ।
लभते गणिकाशब्दं स्थानं च जनसंसदि ।

पूजिता सा सदा राज्ञा गुणवद्भिश्च संस्तुता
प्रार्थनीयाभिगम्या च लक्ष्यभूता च जायते ।

योगज्ञा राजपुत्री च महामात्रसुता तथा
सहस्त्रान्तःपुरमपि स्ववशे कुरुते पतिम् ।

कलानां ग्रहणादेव सौभाग्यमुपजायते ।

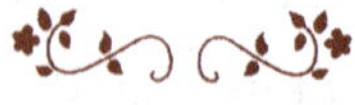

नागरकवृत्त

नगरे पत्तने खर्वटे महति वा सज्जनाश्रये स्थानम्।
यात्रावशाद्वा ।
तत्र भवनमासन्नोदकं वृक्षवाटिकावद्विभक्तकर्मकक्षं
द्विवासगृहं कारयेत् ।

बाह्ये च वासगृहे सुश्लक्ष्णमुभयोपधानं मध्ये विनतं शुक्लोत्तरच्छदं शयनीयं स्यात् । प्रतिशय्यिका च । तस्य शिरोभागे कूर्चस्थानम् वेदिका च। तत्र रात्रिशेषमनुलेपनं माल्यं सिक्थ - करण्डकं सौगन्धिकपुटिका मातुलुङ्गत्वचस्ताम्बूलानि च स्युः । भूमौ पतद्ग्रहः । नागदन्तावसक्ता वीणा । चित्रफलकम् । वर्तिकासमुद्गकः। यः कश्चित्पुस्तकः कुरण्टकमालाश्च । नातिदूरे भूमौ वृत्तास्तरणं समस्तकम् । आकर्षफलकं द्यूतफलकं च । तस्य बहिः क्रीडाशकुनिपञ्जराणि । एकान्ते च तक्षतक्षणस्थान-मन्यासां च क्रीडानाम्। स्वास्तीर्णा प्रेङ्खादोला वृक्षवाटिकायां सप्रच्छाया। स्थंडिलपीठिका च सकुसुमेति भवनविन्यासः ।

स प्रातरुत्थाय कृतनियतकृत्यः, गृहीतदन्तधावनः,
मात्र यानुलेपनं धूपं स्रजमिति च गृहीत्वा,
दत्त्वा सिक्थकमलक्तकं च,
दृष्ट्वा दर्शे मुखम्, गृहीतमुखस वासताम्बूलः, कार्याण्यनुतिष्ठेत् ।

नित्यं स्नानम्। द्वितीयकमुत्सादनम्। तृतीयकः फेनकः। चतुर्थकमायुष्यम्। पञ्चमकं दशमकं वा प्रत्यायुष्यमित्यहीनम्। सातत्याच्च संवृतकक्षास्वेदापनोदः।

पूर्वाह्णापराह्णयोर्भोजनम्। सायं चारायणस्य।

भोजनानन्तरं शुकसारिकाप्रलापनव्यापाराः। लावककुक्कुट-मेषयुद्धानि तास्ताश्च कलाक्रीडाः। पीठमर्दविटविदूषकायत्ता व्यापाराः। दिवाशय्या च।

गृहीतप्रसाधनस्यापराह्णे गोष्ठीविहाराः।

प्रदोषे च संगीतकानि। तदन्ते च प्रसाधिते वासगृहे संचारितसुरभिधूपे ससहायस्य शय्यायाभिसारिकाणां प्रतीक्षणम्।

दूतीनां प्रेषणम्, स्वयं वा गमनम्।

आगतानां च मनोहरैरालापैरुपचारैश्च ससहायस्योपक्रमाः।

घटानिबन्धनम् गोष्ठीसमवायः, समापानकम्, उद्यान गमनम्, समस्याः क्रीडाश्च प्रवर्तयेत्।

पक्षस्य मासस्य वा प्रज्ञातेऽहनि सरस्वत्या भवने नियुक्तानां नित्यं समाजः।
कुशीलवाश्चागन्तवः प्रेक्षणकमेषां दद्युः।

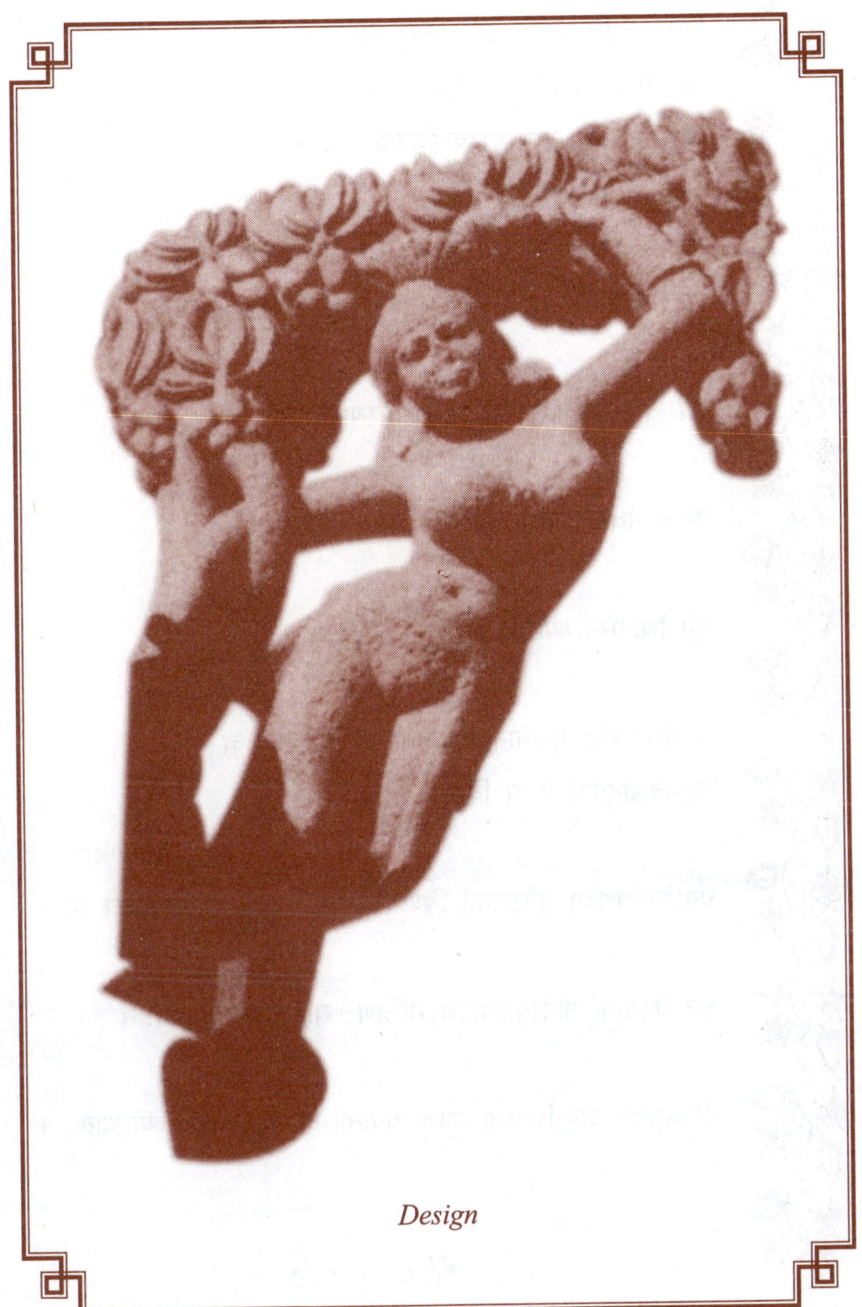

Design

द्वितीयेऽहनि तेभ्यः पूजा नियतं लभेरन्।
ततो यथाश्रद्धमेषां दर्शनमुत्सर्गो वा ।
व्यसनोत्सवेषु चैषां परस्परस्यैककार्यता ।

वेश्याभवने सभायामन्यतमस्योद्वसिते वा समानविद्याबुद्धि-
शीलवित्तयसां सह वेश्याभिरनुरुपैरालापैरासनबन्धो गोष्ठी ।

तत्र चैषां काव्यसमस्या कलासमस्या वा ।

परस्परभवनेषु चापानकानि ।

एतेनोद्यानमनं व्याख्यातम् ।

भुक्तविभवस्तु गुणवान् सकलत्रो वेशे गोष्ठ्यां च
बहुमतस्तदुपजीवी च विटः ।

एकदेशविद्यस्तु क्रीडनको विश्वास्यश्च विदूषकः। वैहासिको वा ।

एते वेश्यानां नागरकाणां च मन्त्रिणः सन्धिविग्रहनियुक्ताः ।

तैर्भिक्षुक्यः कलाविदग्धा मुण्डा वृषल्यो वृद्धगणिकाश्च व्याख्याताः ।

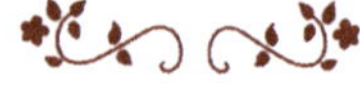

नायकसहायदूतकर्मविमर्श

कामश्चतुर्षु वर्णेषु सवर्णतः शास्त्रतश्चानन्यपूर्वायां प्रयुज्यमानः पुत्रीयो यशस्यो लौकिकश्च भवति।

तद्विपरीत उत्तमवर्णासु परपरिगृहीतासु च ।
प्रतिषिद्धोऽवरवर्णास्वनिरवसितासु ।
वेश्यासु पुनर्भूषु च न शिष्टो न प्रतिषिद्धः । सुखार्थत्वात् ।

तत्र नायिकास्तिस्रः कन्या पुनर्भूर्वेश्या च इति ।

अन्यकारणवशात्परपरिगृहीतापि पाक्षिकी चतुर्थीति गोणिकापुत्रः ।

स यदा मन्यते स्वैरिणीयम् ।

अन्यतोऽपि बहुशो व्यवसितचारित्रा मस्यां वेश्यायामिव गमनमुत्तमवर्णिन्यामपि न धर्मपीडां करिष्यति पुनर्भूरियम् ।

विरसं वा मयि शक्तमपकर्तुकामं च प्रकृतिमापादयिष्यति ।

तया वा मित्रीकृतेन मित्रकार्यममित्रप्रतीघातमन्यद्वा दुष्प्रतिपादकं कार्यं साधयिष्यामि ।

निरत्ययं वास्या गमनमर्थानुबद्धम् । अहं च निःसार-
त्वात्क्षीणवृत्युपायः । सोऽहमनेनोपायेन तद्धनमतिमहदकृच्छ्रा-
दधिागमिष्यामि ।

आयतिमन्तं वा वश्यं पतिं मत्तो विभिद्य द्विषतः संग्राहयिष्यति ।

यामन्यां कामयिष्ये सास्या वशगा ।

तामनेन संक्रमेणाधिगमिष्यामि ।

इति साहसिक्यं न केवलं रागादेव ।

इति परपरिग्रहगमनकारणानि ।

एतैरेव कारणैर्महामात्रसंबद्धा राजसंबद्धा वा तत्रैकदेशचारिणी
काचिदन्या वा कार्यसंपादिनी विधवा पञ्चमीति चारायणः ।

सैव प्रव्रजिता षष्ठीति सुवर्णनाभः ।

गणिकाया दुहिता परिचारिका वानन्यपूर्वा
सप्तमीति घोटकमुखः ।

एक एव तु सार्वलौकिको नायकः । प्रच्छन्नस्तु द्वितीयः ।
विशेषालाभात् । उत्तमाधममध्यमतां तु गुणागुणतो विद्यात् ।
तांस्तूभयोरपि गुणागुणान्वैशिके वक्ष्यामः ।

अगम्यास्त्वेवैताः-कुष्ठिन्युन्मत्ता पतिता भिन्नारहस्या
प्रकाशप्रार्थिनी गतप्राययौवनातिश्वेतातिकृष्णा दुर्गन्धा संब-

न्धिनी सखी प्रव्रजिता संबन्धिसखिश्रोत्रियराजदाराश्च ।

दृष्टपञ्चपुरुषा नागम्या काचिदस्तीति बाभ्रवीयाः ।

सहपांसुक्रीडितमुपकारसम्बद्धं समानशीलव्यसनं सहाध्यायिनं यश्चास्य मर्माणि रहस्यानि च विद्यात्, यस्य चायं विद्याद्वा धात्रपत्यं सहसंवृद्धं मित्रम् ।

रजकनापितमालाकारगान्धिकसौरिकभिक्षुकगोपालकताम्बूलिकसौवर्णिकपीठमर्दविदूषकादयो मित्राणि ।
तद्योषिन्मित्राश्च नागरकाः स्युरिति वात्स्यायनः ।

यदुभयोः साधारणमुभयत्रोदारं विशेषत्तो
नायिकायाः सुविस्त्रब्धं तत्र स्त्रदूतकर्म ।

पटुता धाष्ट्र्यमिङ्गिताकारज्ञता प्रतारणकालज्ञता विषह्य
बुद्धित्वं लघ्वी प्रतिपत्तिः सोपाया चेति दूतगुणाः ।

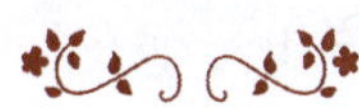

सांप्रयोगिक

रतावस्थापन

शशो वृषोऽश्चइति लिङ्ग.तो नायकविशेषाः ।
नायिका पुनर्मृगी वडवा हस्तिनी चेति ।

तत्र सदृशसंप्रयोगे समरतानि त्रीणि ।

विपर्ययेण विषमाणि षट् । विषमेष्वपि पुरुषाधिक्यं चेद-नन्तरसंप्रयोगे द्वे उच्चरते । व्यवहितमेकमुच्चतररतम् । विपर्यये पुनर्द्वे नीचरते । व्यवहितमेकं नीचतररतं च । तेषु समानि श्रेष्ठानि । तरशब्दाङ्किते द्वे कनिष्ठा । शेषाणि मध्यमानि ।

साम्येऽप्युच्चाङ्गाज्ज्यायः । इति प्रमाणतो नवरतानि ।

यस्य संप्रयोगकाले प्रीतिरुदासीना वीर्यमल्पं क्षतानि च
न सहते स मन्दवेगः ।

तद्विपर्ययौ मध्यमचण्डवेगौ भवतः । तथा नायिकापि ।

तत्रापि प्रमाणवदेव नवरतानि ।

तद्वत्कालतोऽपि शीघ्रमध्यचिरकाला नायकाः ।

तत्र स्त्रियां विवादः ।

न स्त्री पुरुषवदेव भावमधिगच्छति ।

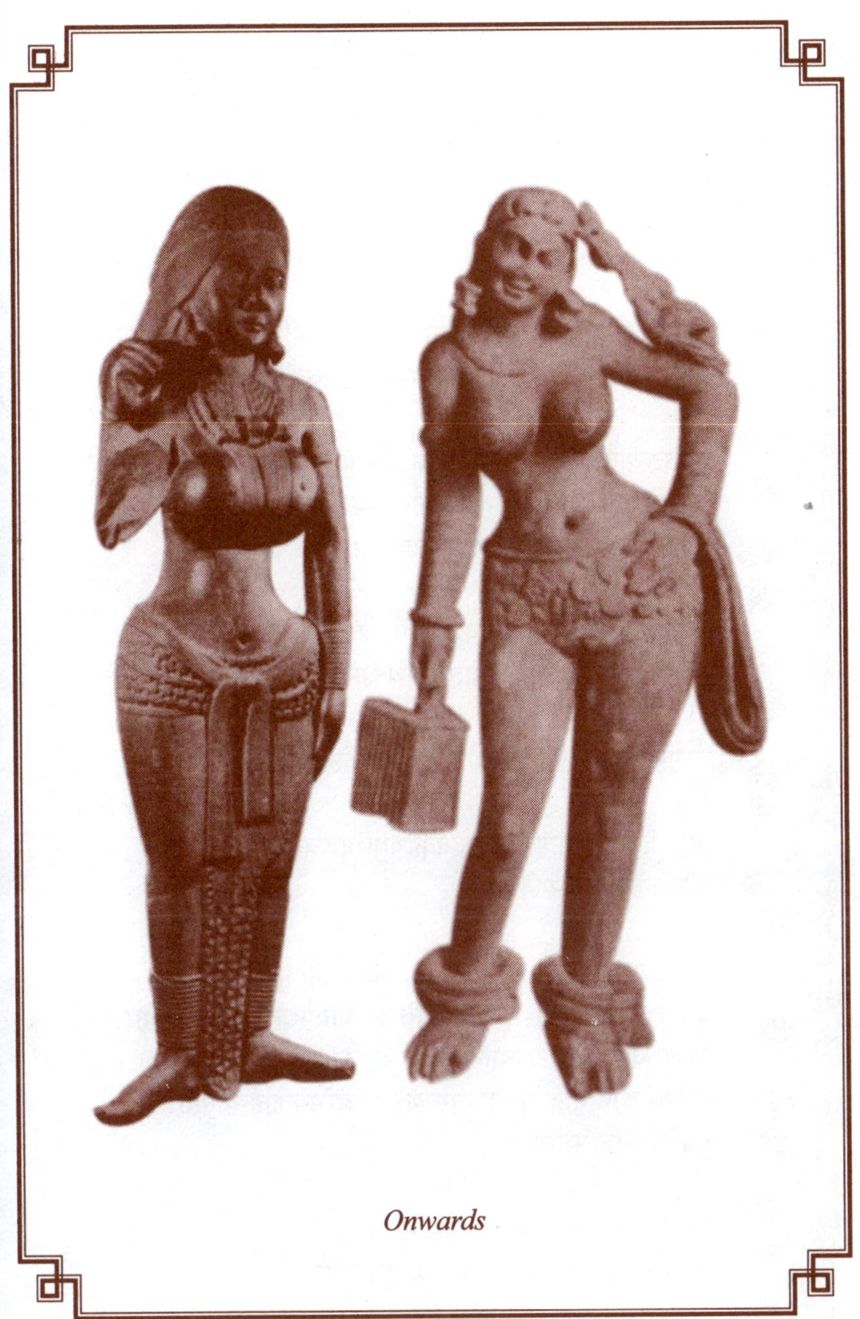

Onwards

सातत्यात्त्वस्याः पुरुषेण कण्डूतिरपनुद्यते ।

सा पुनराभिमानिकेन सुखेन संसृष्टा रसान्तरं जनयति तस्मिन् सुखबुद्धिरस्याः ।

पुरुषप्रीतेश्चानभिज्ञत्वात्कथं ते सुखमिति प्रष्टुमशक्यत्वात् ।

कथमेतदुपलभ्यत इति चेत्पुरुषो हि रतिमधिगम्य स्वेच्छयाविरमति, न स्त्रियमपेक्षते, न त्वेवं स्त्रीत्यौद्दालकिः ।

तत्रैतत्स्यात् । चिरवेगे, नायके स्त्रियोऽनुरज्यन्ते, शीघ्रवेगस्य भावमनासाद्यावसानेऽभ्यसूयिन्यो भवन्ति । तत्सर्वं भावप्राप्तेरप्राप्तेश्च लक्षणम् ।

तञ्च न । कण्डूतिप्रतीकारोऽपि हि दीर्घकालं प्रिय इति । एतदुपपद्यत एव । तस्मात्संदिग्धत्वादलक्षणमिति ।

तस्मात्पुरूषवदेव योषितोऽपि रसव्यक्तिर्द्रष्टव्या ।

कथं हि समानायामेवाकृतावेकार्थमभिप्रपन्नयोः कार्यवैल क्षण्यंस्यात् ।

कथमुपायवैलक्षण्यं तु सर्गात् । कर्ता हि पुरुषोऽधिकरणं युवतिः । अन्यथा हि कर्ता क्रियां प्रतिपद्यतेऽन्यथा चाधारः । तस्माच्चोपायवैलक्षण्यात्सर्गादभिमानवैलक्षण्यमपि भवति । अभियोक्ताहमिति पुरुषोऽनुरज्यते । अभियुक्ताहमनेनेति युवतिरितिवात्स्यायनः ।

जातेरभद्दाम्पत्योः सदृशं सुखमिष्यते । तस्मात्तथोपचर्या स्त्री यथाग्रे प्राप्नुयाद्रतिम् ।

प्रथमरते चण्डवेगता शीघ्रकालता च पुरुषस्य,
तद्विपरीतमुत्तरेषु । योषितः पुनरेतदेव विपरीतम् ।
आ धातुक्षयात् ।

अभ्यासादभिमानाञ्च तथा संप्रत्ययादपि ।
विषयभ्येश्च तन्त्रज्ञाः प्रीतिमाहुश्चतुर्विधाम् ।

शब्दादिभ्यो बहिर्भूता या कर्माभ्यासलक्षणा ।
प्रीतिः साभ्यासिकी ज्ञेया मृगयादिषु कर्मसु ।

अनभ्यस्तेष्वपि पुरा कर्मस्वविषयात्मिका ।
संकल्पाञ्जायते प्रीतिर्या सा स्यादाभिमानिकी ।

प्रकृतेर्या तृतीयस्याः स्त्रियाश्चैवोपरिष्टके ।
तेषु तेषु च विज्ञेया चुम्बनादिषु कर्मसु ।

नान्योऽयमिति यत्र स्यादन्यस्मिन्प्रीतिकारणे ।
तन्त्रज्ञैः कथ्यते सापि प्रीतिः संप्रत्ययात्मिका ।

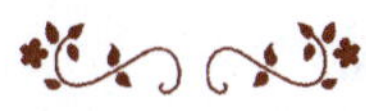

आलिङ्गन

आलिङ्ग.नचुम्बननखच्छेद्यदशनच्छेद्यसंवेशनसीत्कृतपुरुषायि-
तौपरिष्टकानामष्टानामष्टधा
विकल्पभेदादष्टाकाश्चतु:षष्टिरिति वाभ्रवीया: ।

विकल्पवर्गाणामष्टानां न्यूनाधिकत्वदर्शनात् प्रहणनविरुत-
पुरुषोपसृप्तचित्ररतादीनामन्येषामपि वर्गाणामिह प्रवेशनात्प्रायो-
वादोऽयम् । यथा सप्तपर्णो वृक्ष: पञ्चवर्णो बलिरिति वात्स्यायन: ।

तत्रासमागतयो: प्रीतिलिङ्ग.द्योतनार्थमालिङ्ग.नचतुष्टयम् ।
स्पृष्टकम्, विद्धकम्, उद्घृष्टकम्, पीडितकम्, इति ।

संमुखागतायां प्रयोज्यायामन्यापदेशेन गच्छतो
गात्रेण गात्रस्य स्पर्शनं स्पृष्टकम् ।

प्रयोज्यं स्थितमुपविष्टं वा विजने किंचिद् गृह्णती पयोधरेण
विध्येत। नायकोऽपि तामवपीड्य गृह्णीयादिति विद्धकम् ।

तदुभयमनतिप्रवृत्तसंभाषणयो: ।

तमसि जनसंबाधे विजने वाथ शनकैर्गच्छतोर्नातिह्रस्व-

क्षलमुद्वर्पणं परस्परस्य गात्राणामुद्घृष्टकम् ।

तदेव कुड्यसंदंशेन वा स्फुटकमवपीडयेदिति पीडितकम् ।

तदुभयमवगतपरस्पराकारयोः ।

लतावेष्टितकं वृक्षाधिरूढकं तिलतण्डुलकं
क्षीरनीरकमिति चत्वारि संप्रयोगकाले ।

लतेव शालमावेष्टयन्ती चुम्बनार्थं मुखमवनमयेत् । उद्धृत्य
मन्दसीत्कृता तमाश्रिता वा किंचिद्रामणीयकं पश्येत्तल्लतावेष्टितकम् ।

चरणेन चरणमाक्रम्य द्वितीयेनोरुदेशमाक्रमन्ती वेष्टयन्ती वा
तत्पृठष्सक्तैकबाहुर्द्वितीयेनांसमवनमयन्ती ईषन्मन्दसीत्कृतकूजिता
चुम्बनार्थमेवाधिरोढुमिच्छेदिति वृक्षाधिरूढकम् ।

तदुभयं स्थितकर्म ।

शयनगतावेवोरुव्यत्यासं भुजव्यत्यासं च ससंघर्षमिव
घनं संस्वजेते तत्तिलतण्डुलकम् ।

रागान्धावनपेक्षितात्ययौ परस्परमनुविशत
इवोत्सङ्ग.गतायामभिमुखोपविष्टायां शयने वेति क्षीरजलकम् ।

तदुभयं रागकाले ।
सुवर्णनाभस्य त्वधिकमेकाङ्ग.ोपगूहनचतुष्टयम् ।

त्रयोरूसंदर्शेनकैमूरूमूरूद्वयं
वा सर्वप्राणं पीडयेदित्यूरूपगूहनम्

जघनेन जघनमवपीड्य प्रकीर्यमाणकेशहस्ता नखदशनप्रहण-
नचुम्बनप्रयोजनाय तदुपरि लंघयेत्तज्ञघनोपगूहनम् ।

स्तनाभ्यामुरः प्रविश्य तत्रैव भारमारोपयेदिति स्तनालिङ्ग.नम् ।

मुखे मुखमासज्याक्षिणी अक्ष्णोर्ललाटेन
ललाटमाहन्यात्सा ललाटिका ।
संवाहनमप्युपगूहनप्रकारमित्येके मन्यन्ते ।
संस्पर्शत्वाद् ।

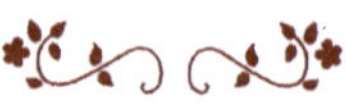

चुम्बन

चुम्बननखदशनच्छेद्यानां न पौर्वापर्यमस्ति ।
रागयोगात् प्राक्संयोगादेषां प्राधान्येन प्रयोगः।
प्रहणनसीत्कृतयोश्च संप्रयोगे ।

ललाटालककपोलनयनवक्षःस्तनोष्ठान्तर्मुखेषु चुम्बनम् ।

ऊरुसंधिबाहुनाभिमूलयोर्लाटानाम् ।

तद्यथा-निमित्तकं स्फुरितकं घट्टितकमिति
त्रीणि कन्या चुम्बनानि ।

बलात्कारेण नियुक्ता मुखे मुखमाधत्ते न तु
विचेष्टत इति निमित्तकम् ।

वदने प्रवेशितं चौष्ठं मनागपत्रपावग्रहीतुमिच्छन्ती
स्पन्दयति स्वमोष्ठं नोत्तरमुत्सहत इति स्फुरितकम् ।

ईषत्परिगृह्य विनिमीलितनयना करेण च तस्य नयने
अवच्छादयन्ती जिह्वाग्रेण घट्टयति इति घट्टितकम् ।

समं तिर्यगुद्भान्तमवपीडितकमिति चतुर्विधमपरे ।

अङ्गुलिसंपुटेन पिण्डीकृत्य निर्दशनमोष्ठपुटेनावपीडयेदि त्यवपीडितकं पञ्चममपि करणम् ।

द्यूतं चात्र प्रवर्तयेत् ।

पूर्वमधरसंपादनेन जितमिदं स्यात् ।

तत्र जिता सार्धरुदितं करं विधुनुयात्प्रणुदेद्दशेत्परिवतं-
येद्धलादाहृता विवदेज्पुनरप्यस्तु पण इति ब्रूयात् ।
तत्रापि जिता द्विगुणमायस्येत् ।

विश्रब्धस्य प्रमतस्य वाधरमवगृह्य दशनान्तर्गतमनिर्गमं कृत्वा
हसेदुत्क्रोशेत्तर्जयेद्वल्गेदाह्वयेन्नृत्येत्प्रनर्तितभ्रुणा च
विचलनयनेन मुखेन विहसन्ती तानि तानि च ब्रूयात् ।
इति चुंम्बन द्यूतकलहः ।

एतेन नखदशनच्छेद्यप्रहणनद्यूजकलहा व्याख्याताः ।

तस्यां चुम्बन्त्यामयमप्युत्तरं गृह्णीयात् । इत्युत्तरचुम्बितम् ।

ओष्ठसंदंशेनावगृह्यौष्ठद्वयमपि चुम्बते । इति संपुटकं स्त्रियाः,
पुंसो वाऽजातव्यञ्जनस्य ।

तस्मिन्नितरोऽपि जिह्वयास्या दशनान्घट्टयेतालु जिह्वां चेति जिह्वायुद्धम् ।

एतेन बलाद्वदनरदनग्रहणं दानं च व्याख्यातम् ।

समं पीडितमञ्चितं मृदु शेषाङ्गे.षु चुम्बनं स्थानविशेषयोगात् ।
इति चुम्बनविशेषाः ।

सुप्तस्य मुखमवलोकयन्त्या स्वाभिप्रायेण चुम्बनं राग दीपनम् ।

प्रमत्तस्य विवदमानस्य वाऽन्यतोऽभिमुखस्य
सुप्ताभिमुखस्य वा निद्राव्याघातार्थ चलितकम् ।

चिररात्रावागतस्य शयनसुप्तायाः स्वाभिप्रायचुम्बनं
प्रातिबोधिकम् ।

आदर्शे कुड्ये सलिले वा प्रयोज्यायारछायाचुम्बनमाकार
प्रदर्शनार्थमेव कार्यम् ।

बालस्य चित्रकर्मणः प्रतिमायाश्च चुम्बनं
संक्रान्तकमालिङ्ग.नं च ।

कृते प्रतिकृतं कुर्यात्ताडिते प्रतिताडितम् ।
करणेन च तेनैव चुम्बिते प्रतिचुम्बितम् ।

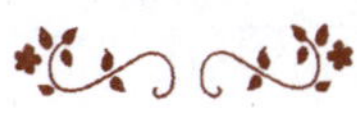

नखरदन

रागवृद्धौ संघर्षात्मकं नखविलेखनम् ।

तथा दशनच्छेद्यस्य सात्म्यवशाद्वा ।

तदाच्छुरितकमर्धचन्द्रो मण्डलं रेखा व्याघ्रनखं मयूरपदकं शशप्लुतकमुत्पलपत्रकमिति रूपतोऽष्टविकल्पम् ।

कक्षौ स्तनौ गलः पृष्ठं जघनमूरू च स्थानानि ।

प्रवृत्तरतिचक्राणां न स्थानमस्थानं वा विद्यत इति सुवर्णनाभः ।

तत्र सव्यहस्तानि प्रत्यग्रशिखराणि द्वित्रिशिखराणि चण्डवेगयोर्नखानि स्युः ।

अनुगतराजि सममुज्ज्वलममलिनमविपाटितं विवर्धिष्णु मृदुस्निग्धदर्शनमिति नखगुणाः ।

दीर्घाणि हस्तशोभीन्यालोके च योषितां चितग्राहीणि गौडानां नखानि स्युः ।

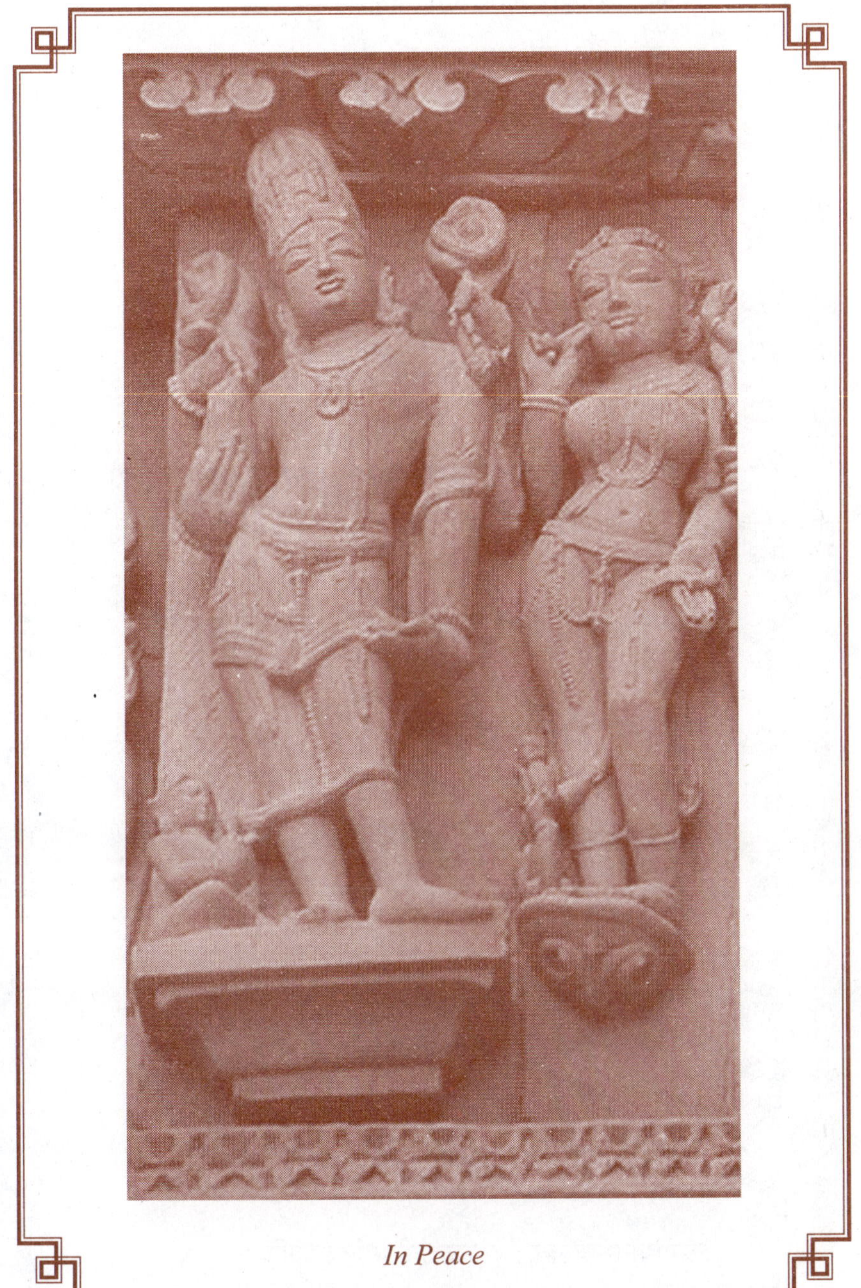

In Peace

ह्रस्वानि कर्मसहिष्णूनि विकल्पयोजनासु च स्वेच्छापातीनि दाक्षिणात्यानाम् ।

मध्यमान्युभयभाञ्जि महाराष्ट्रकाणामिति ।

तैः सुनियमितैर्हनुदेशो स्तनयोरधरे वा लघुकरणमनुग्तलेखं स्पर्शमात्रजननाद्रोमाञ्चकरमन्ते संनिपावर्धमानशब्दमाच्छुरितकम् ।

प्रयोज्यायां च तस्याङ्ग.संवाहने शिरसः कण्डूयने पिटकभेदने व्याकुलीकरणे भीषणेन प्रयोगः ।

ग्रीवायां: स्तनपृष्ठे च वक्रो नखपदनिवेशोऽर्धचन्द्रकः ।

तावेव द्वौ परस्पराभिमुखौ मण्डलम् ।

नाभिमूलककुन्दरवंक्षणेषु तस्य प्रयोगः ।

सर्वस्थानेषु नातिदीर्घा लेखा ।

सैव वक्रा व्याघ्रनखकमास्तनमुखम् ।

पञ्चभिरभिमुखैर्लेखा चूचुकाभिमुखी मयूरपदकम् ।

तत्संप्रयोगश्लाघायाः स्तनचूचुके संनिकृष्टानि

पञ्चनखपदानि शशाप्लुतकम् ।

स्तनपृष्ठे मेखलापथे चोत्पलपत्रकृतीत्युत्पलपत्रकम् ।

ऊर्वोः स्तनपृष्ठे च प्रवासं गच्छतः स्मारणीयकं
संहताश्चतस्त्रस्तिस्त्रो वा लेखाः ।

आकृतिविकारयुक्तानि चान्यान्यपि कुर्वीत ।

भवति हि रागेऽपि चित्रापेक्षा । वैचित्र्याच्च परस्परं
रागो जनयितव्यः । वैचक्षण्ययुक्ताश्च गणिकास्तत्कामिनश्च
परस्परं प्रार्थनीया भवन्ति । धनुर्वेदादिष्वपि हि शस्त्रकर्मशास्त्रेषु
वैचित्र्य मेवापेक्ष्यते किं पुनरिहेतिवात्स्यायनः ।

न तु परपरिगृहीतास्वेवं कुर्यात् । प्रच्छन्नेषु
प्रदशेषु तासामनुस्मरणार्थं रागवर्धनाच्च विशेषान्दर्शयेत् ।

नखक्षतानि पश्यन्त्या गूढस्थानेषु योषितः ।
चिरोत्सृष्टाप्यभिनवा प्रीतिर्भवति पेशला ।

नान्यत्पटुतरं किंचिदस्ति रागविवर्धनम् ।
नखदन्तसमुत्थानां कर्मणां गतयो यथा ।

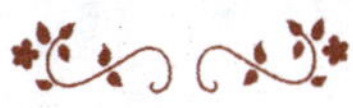

दशनच्छेद्य

उतरौष्ठमन्तर्मुखं नयनमिति मुक्त्वा
चुम्बनवद्दशनरदनस्थानानि ।

समाः स्निग्धच्छाया रागग्राहिणो युक्तप्रमाणा
निश्छिद्रास्तीक्ष्णाग्रा इति दशनगुणाः ।

कुण्ठा राज्युद्गताः परुषाः विषमाः श्लक्ष्णाः
पृथवो विरला इति च दोषाः ।

गूढकमुच्छूनकं बिन्दुर्बिन्दुमाला प्रवालमणिर्मणिमाला
खण्डाभ्रकं वराहचर्वितकमिति दशनच्छेदनविकल्पाः ।

नातिलोहितेन रागमात्रेण विभावनीयं गूढकम् ।

तदेव पीडनादुच्छूनकम् ।

तदुभयं बिन्दुरधरमध्य इति ।

उच्छूनकं प्रवालमणिश्च कपोले ।

कर्णपूरचुम्बनं नखदशनच्छेद्यमिति सव्यकपोलमण्डनानि ।

दन्तौष्ठसंयोगाभ्यासनिष्पादनात्प्रवालमणिसिद्धिः ।

सर्वस्येयं मणिमालायाश्च ।

अल्पदेशायाश्च त्व चो दशनद्वयसंदंशजा बिन्दुसिद्धिः । सर्वैर्बिन्दुमालायाश्च ।

तस्मान्मालाद्वयमपि गलकक्षवंक्षणप्रदेशेषु ।

ललाटे चोर्वोर्बिन्दुमाला ।

मण्डलमिव विषमकूटकयुक्तं खण्डाभ्रकं स्तनपृष्ठ एव।

संहताः प्रदीर्घा बह्वयो दशनपदराजयस्ताम्रान्तराला वराहचर्वितकम् । स्तनपृष्ठ एव ।

तदुभयमपि च चण्डयवेगयोः ।

मध्यदेश्या आर्यप्राया: शुच्युपचाराश्चुम्बननखदन्तपदद्वेषिण्यः ।

बाह्लीकदेश्या आवन्तिकाश्च ।

चित्ररतेषु त्वासामभिनिवेशः ।

परिष्वङ्ग.चुम्बननखदन्तचूषणप्रधानाः क्षतवर्जिताः
प्रहणनसाध्या मालव्य आभीर्यश्च ।

सिन्धुषष्ठानां च नदीनामन्तरालीया औपरिष्टकसात्म्याः ।

चण्डवेगा मन्दासीत्कृता आपरान्तिका लाट्यश्च ।

दृढप्रहणनयोगिन्यः खरवेगा एव, अपद्रव्यप्रधानाः
स्त्रीराज्ये कोशलायां च ।

प्रकृत्या मृद्व्यो रतिप्रिया अशुचिरुचयो निराचाराश्चान्ध्रयः ।

सकलचतुःषष्टिप्रयोगरागिण्योऽश्लीलपरुषवाक्यप्रियाः
शयने च सरभसोपक्रमा महाराष्ट्रिकाः ।

तथाविधा एव रहसि प्रकाशन्ते नागरिकाः ।

मृद्यमानाश्चाभियोगान्मन्दं मन्दं प्रसिञ्चन्ते द्रविड्यः ।

मध्यमवेगाः सर्वसहाः स्वाङ्ग.प्रच्छादिन्यः पराङ्ग.हासिन्यः

कुत्सिताश्लीलपरुषपरिहारिण्यो वानवासिकाः ।

मृदुभाषिण्र्याऽनुरागवत्यो मृद्वयङ्गयश्च गौड्यः
वार्यमाणश्च पुरुषो यत्कुर्यात्तदनु क्षतम् ।
अमृष्माणा द्विगुणं तदेव प्रतियोजयेत् ।

बिन्दोः प्रतिक्रिया माला मालायाश्चाभ्रखण्डकम् ।
इति क्रोधादिवाविष्टा कलहान्प्रतियोजयेत् ।

परस्परानुकूल्येन तदेवं लज्जमानयोः ।
संवत्सरशतेनापि प्रीतिर्न परिहीयते ।

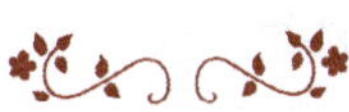

संवेशन

रागकाले विशालयन्त्येव जघनं मृगी संविशेदुच्चरते ।

अवह्रासयन्तीव हस्तिनी नीचरते ।

न्याय्यो यत्र योगस्तत्र समपृष्ठम् ।

आभ्यां वडवा व्याख्याता ।

तत्र जघनेन नायकं प्रतिगृह्णीयात् ।

अपद्रव्याणि च सविशेषं नीचरते ।

उत्फुल्लकं विजृम्भितकमिन्द्राणिकं चेति त्रितयं
मृग्याः प्रायेण ।

शिरो विनिपात्योर्ध्वं जघनमुत्फुल्लकम् ।

तत्रापसारं दद्यात् ।

अनीचे सक्थिनी तिर्यगवसज्य प्रतीच्छेदिति विजृम्भितकम् ।

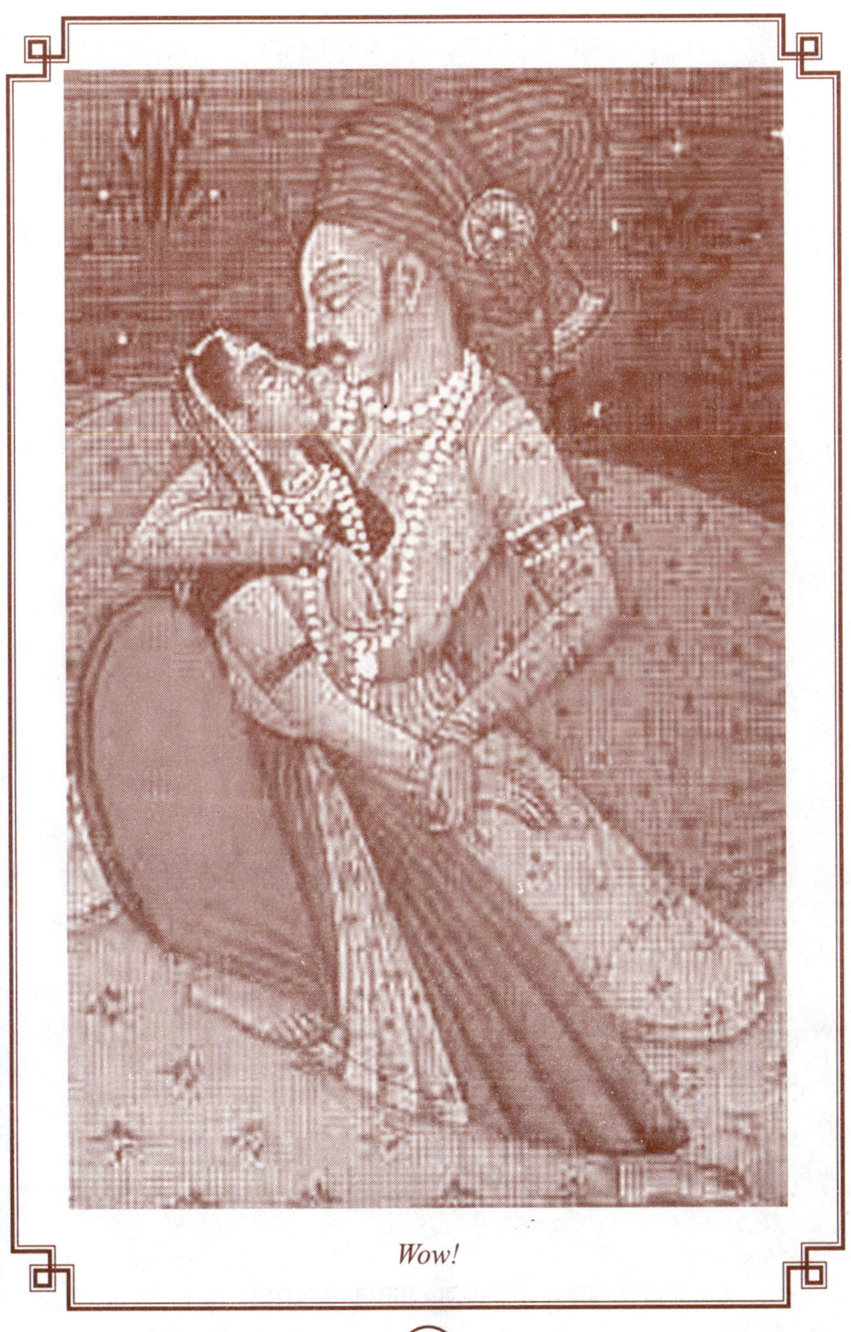

Wow!

पार्श्वयोः सममूरू विन्यस्य पार्श्वयोर्जानुनी निदध्यादित्यभ्यासयोगादिन्द्राणी ।

त्योच्चतररतस्यापि परिग्रहः ।

संपुटेन प्रतिग्रहो नीचरते ।

एतेन नीचतररतेऽपि हस्तिन्याः ।

संपुटकं पीडितकं वेष्टिकं वाडवकमिति ।

ऋजुप्रसारितावुभावप्युभयोश्चरणाविति संपुटः ।

स द्विविधः पार्श्वसंपुट उत्तसंपुटश्च । तथा कर्मयोगात् ।

पार्श्वेण तु शयानो दक्षिणेन नारीमधिशयीतेति सार्वत्रिकमेतत् ।

संपुटकप्रयुक्तयन्त्रेणैव दृढमूरू पीडयेदिति पीडितकम् ।

ऊरू व्यत्यस्येदिति वेष्टितकम् ।

वडवेव निष्ठुरमर्थंगृह्णीयादिति वाडवकमाभ्यासिकम् ।

तदान्ध्रीषु प्रायेण । इति संवेशनप्रकारा बाभ्रवीयाः ।

सौवर्णनाभास्तु ।

उभावप्यूरू ऊर्ध्वाविति तभ्दुग्नकम् ।

चराणावूर्ध्वं नायकोऽस्या धारयेदिति जृम्भितकम् ।

तत्कुञ्चितावुत्पीडितकम् ।

तदेकस्मिन्प्रसारितेऽर्धपीडितकम् ।

नायकस्यांस एको द्वितीयकः प्रसारित इति पुनः
पुनर्व्यत्यासेन वेणुदारितकम् ।

एकः शिरस उपरि गच्छेद्वितीयः प्रसारित
इति शूलाचितकमाभ्यासिकम् ।

संकुचितौ स्वस्तिदेशो निदध्यादिति कार्कटकम् ।

ऊर्ध्वावूरू व्यत्यस्येदिति पीडितकम् ।

जङ्घाव्यत्यासेन पद्मासनवत् ।
पृष्ठं परिष्वजमानायाः पराङ्मुखेण परावृत्तकमाभ्यासिकम् ।
जले च संविष्टोपविष्टस्थितात्मकांश्चित्रान्योगानुपलक्षयेत् ।
तथा सुकरत्वादिति सुवर्णनाभः ।

वार्तं तु तत् । शिष्टैरपस्मृतत्वादिति वात्स्यायनः ।

अथ चित्ररतानि ।

ऊर्ध्वस्तियोर्यूनोः परस्परापाश्रययोः
कुड्यस्तम्भापाश्रितयोर्वा स्थितरतम् ।

कुड्याचापाश्रितस्य कण्ठावसक्तबाहुपाशायास्तद्धस्तपञ्जरो
पविष्टाया ऊरुपाशेन जघनमभिवेष्टयन्त्या कुड्ये
चरणक्रमेण वलन्त्या अवलम्बितकं रतम् ।

भूमौ वा चतुज़्पदवदास्थिताया वृषलीयावस्किन्दनं धेनुकम् ।

तत्र पृष्ठमुरःकर्माणि लभते ।
एतेनैव योगेन शौनमैणेयं छागलं गर्दभाक्रान्तं मार्जार-
ललितकं व्याघ्रावस्कन्दनं गजोपमर्दितं वराहघृष्टकं तुरगाधिरूढ-
कमिति यत्र यत्र विशेषो योगोऽपूर्वस्तत्तदुपलक्षयेत् ।

मिश्रीकृतसद्भावाभ्यां द्वाभ्यां सह संघाटकं रतम् ।

बह्वीभिश्च सह गोयूथिकम् ।
वारिक्रीडितकं छागलमैणेयमिति तत्कर्मानुकृतियोगात् ।

ग्रामनारीविषये स्त्रीराज्ये च बाह्लीके बहवो युवानोऽन्तः ।

पुरसधर्माण एकैकस्याः परिग्रहभृताः ।

तेषामेकैकशो युगपच्च यथासात्म्यं यथायोगं च रञ्जयेयुः ।

अधोरतं पायावपि दाक्षिणात्यानाम् ।

तत्सात्म्याद्देशसात्म्याच्च तैस्तैर्भावैः प्रयोजितैः ।
स्त्रीणां स्नेहश्च रागश्च बहुमानश्च जायते ।

पुरुषायित

नायकस्य संतताभ्यासात्परिश्रममुपलभ्य रागस्य चानुपशमम्, अनुमता तेन तमधोऽवपात्य पुरुषायितेन साहाय्यं दद्यात् ।

स्वाभिप्रायाद्वा विकल्पयोजनार्थिनी ।

नायककुतूहलाद्वा ।

सा प्रकीर्यमाणकेशकुसुमा श्वासविच्छिहासिनी वक्त्र-संसर्गार्थं स्तनाभ्यामुरः पीडयन्ती पुनः पुनः शिरो नामयन्ती याश्चेष्टाः पूर्वमसौ दर्शितवांस्ता एव प्रतिकुर्वीत । पातिता प्रतिपातयामीति हसन्ती तर्जयन्ती प्रतिघ्नती च ब्रूयात् । पुनश्च व्रीडां दर्शयेत् । श्रमं विरामाभीप्सां च । पुरुषोपसृप्तैरेवोपसर्पेत् ।

वरणसंविधान

सवर्णायामनन्यपूर्वायां शास्त्रतोऽधिगतायां धर्मोऽर्थः पुत्राः संबन्धः पक्षवृद्धिरनुपस्कृता रतिश्च ।

तस्मात्कन्यामभिजनोपेतां मातापितृमतीं त्रिवर्षात्प्रभृति न्यूनवयसं श्लाघ्याचारे धनवति पक्षवति कुले संबन्धिप्रिये संबन्धिभिराकुले प्रसूतां प्रभूतमातृपितृपक्षां रूपशीललक्षणसंपन्ना-मन्यूनसाधिकाविनष्टदन्तनखकर्णकेशाक्षिस्तनीमरोगिप्रकृतिशरीरां तथाविध एव श्रुतवाञ्शीलयेत् ।

यां गृहीत्वा कृतिमात्मानं मन्येत न च समानैर्निन्द्येत तस्यां प्रवृत्तिरिति घोटकमुखः ।

तदेतद् ब्रह्मचर्येण परेण च समाधिना ।
विहितं लोकयात्राऽर्थं न रागार्थोऽस्य संविधिः ।

रक्षन्धर्मार्थकामानां स्थितिं स्वां लोकवर्तिनीम् ।
अस्य शास्त्रस्य तत्त्वज्ञो भवत्येव जितेन्द्रियः ।

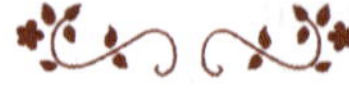

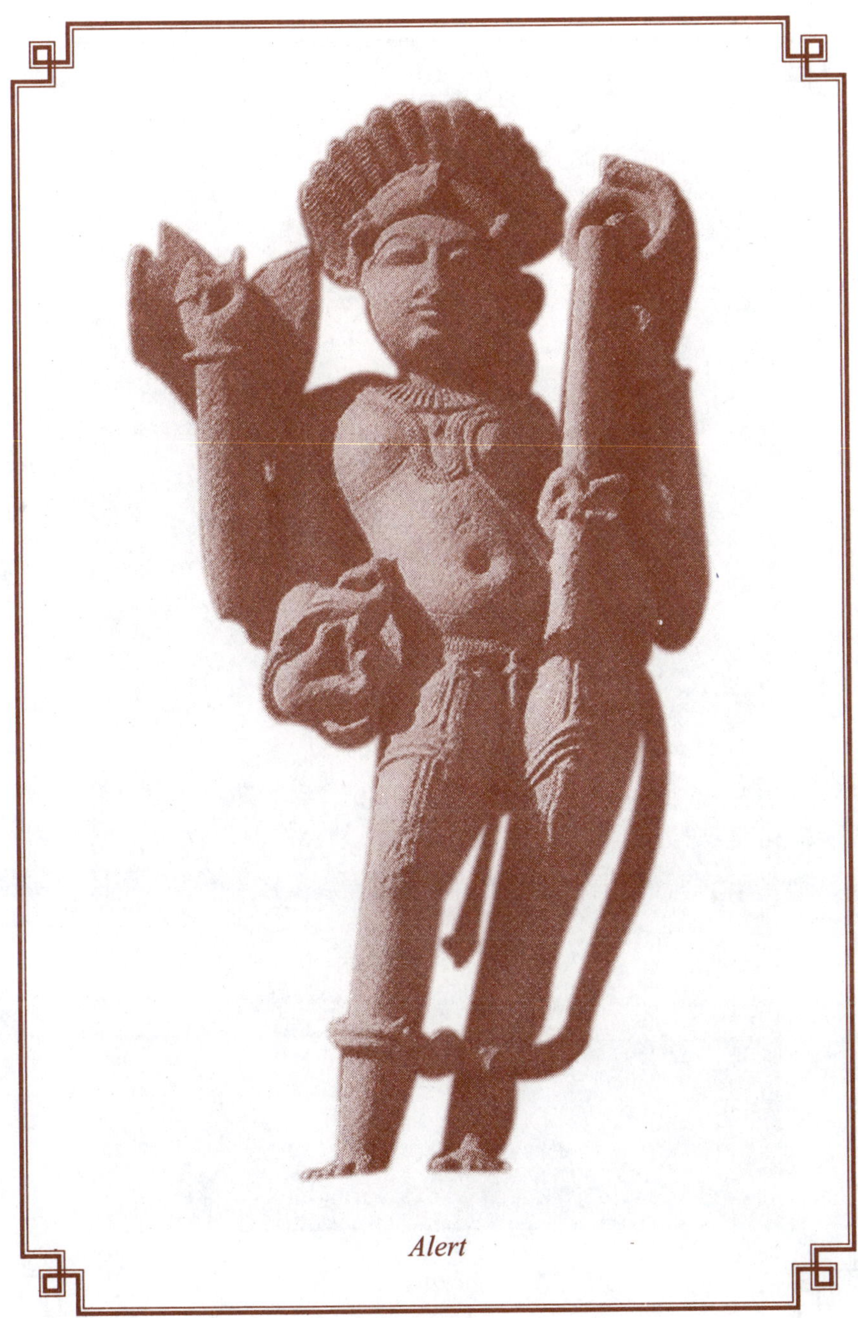

Alert

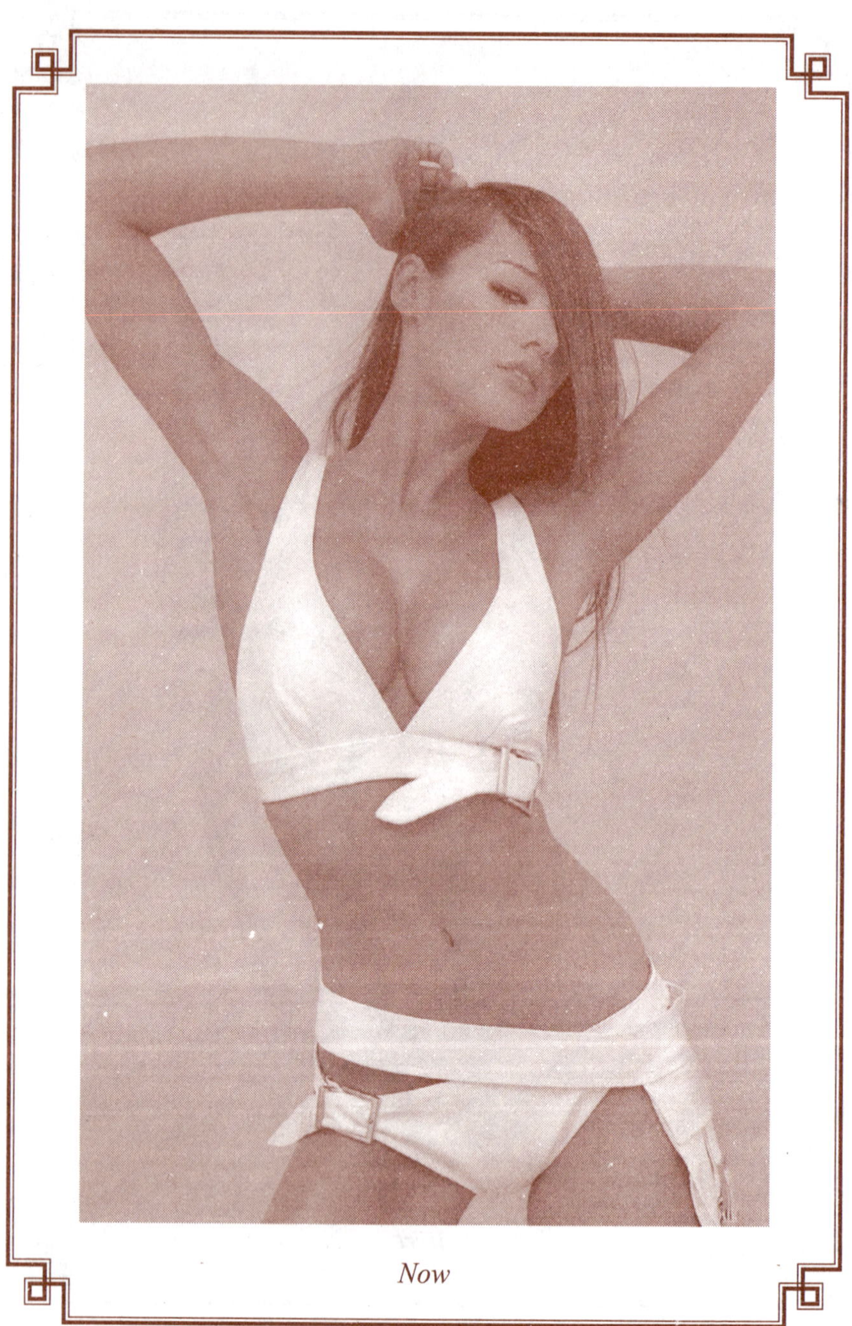

Now

The Kamasutra

English Translation by Sir Richard Burton and F. F. Arbuthnot

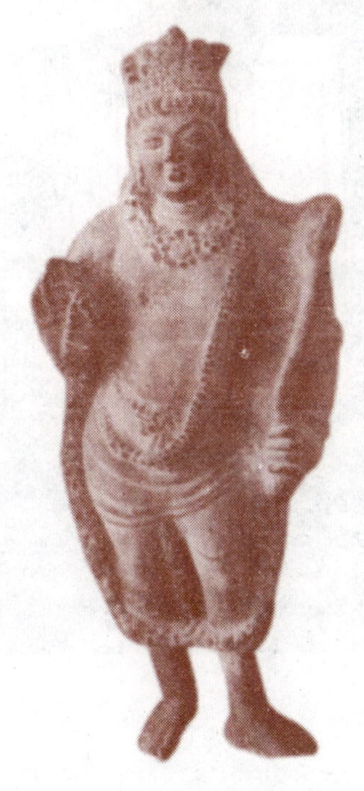

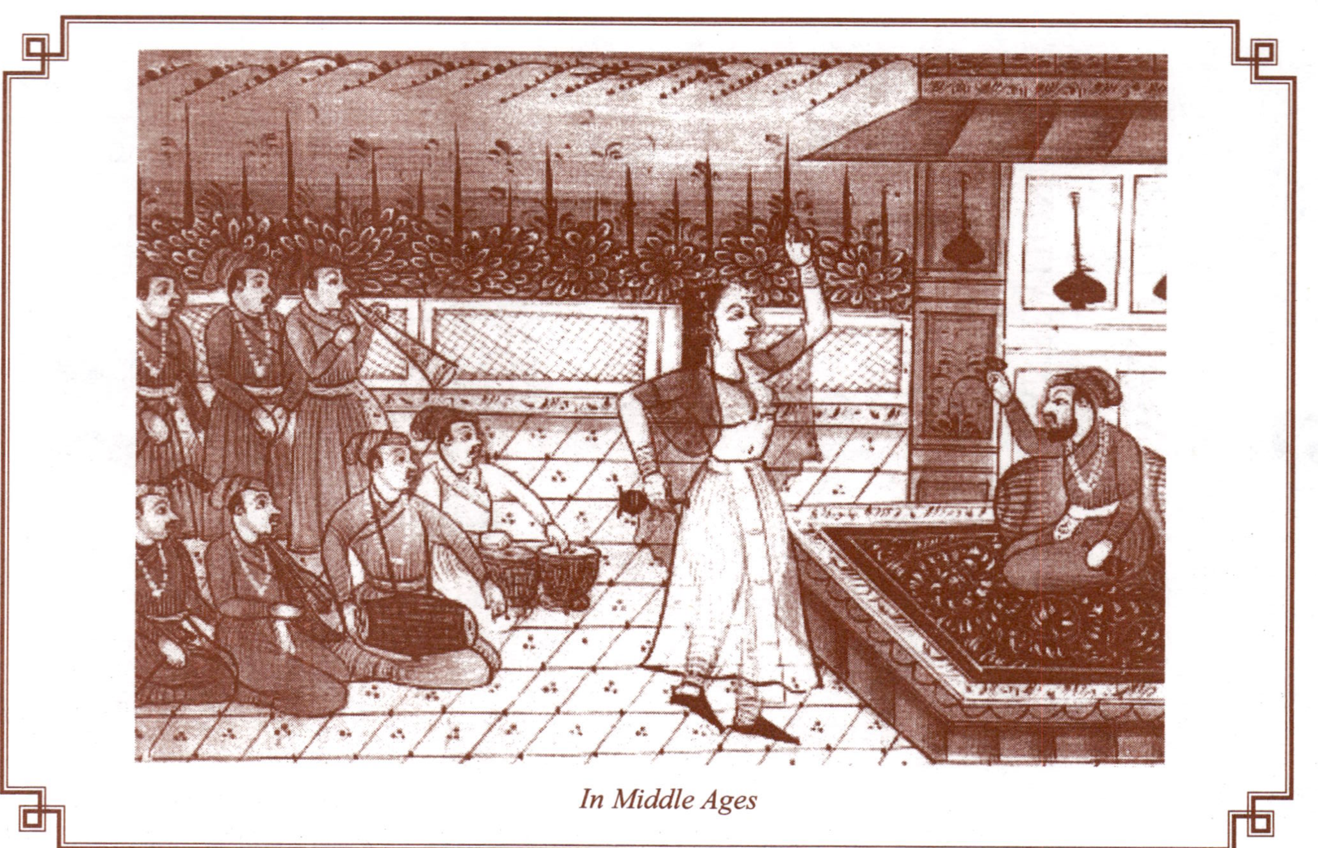

In Middle Ages

1

KAMA IN HUMAN LIFE

Man whose life is one hundred years should practice Dharma, Artha and Kama at different times and in such a manner that they may harmonize together and not clash in any way.

He should acquire learning in his childhood, in his youth and in his middle age he should attend to Artha and Kama and in his old age he should perform Dharma, and thus seek to gain Moksha, the release from further transmigration, or, on account of uncertainty of life he may practise them at times when they are enjoined to be practised. But one thing is to be noted, he should lead the life of a religious student until he finishes his education.

Dharma is obedience to the command of the Shastra of the Hindus to do certain things, such as performance of sacrifices, which are not generally done. Because they do not belong to this world, and produce no visible effect; and not to do other things, such as eating meat, which is often done because it belongs to this world and has visible effects.

Dharma should be learnt from Shruti and from those conversant with it.

Artha is the acquisition of arts, land, gold, cattle, wealth, equipages and friends. It is further the protection

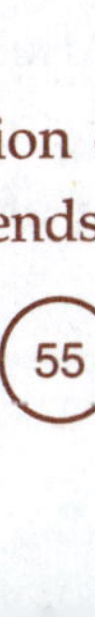

of what is acquired and the increase of what is protected.

Artha should be learnt from king's officers, and from merchants who may be versed in the ways of commerce.

Kama is the enjoyment of appropriate objects by the five senses of hearing, feeling, seeing, tasting and smelling, assisted by the mind together with the soul. The ingredient in this is a peculiar contact between the organ of sense and its object, and the consciousness of pleasure which arises from that contact is called Kama.

Kama is to be learnt from the Kamasutra and from the practice of citizens.

Thus I have written in a few words the 'Science of Love', after reading the text of ancient authors, and following the ways of enjoyment mentioned in them.

He who is acquainted with the true principles of the science pays regard to Dharma, Artha, and to its own experiences, as well as to the teaching of others and does not act simply on the dictates of his own desires. As for the errors in the science of love which I have mentioned in this work, on my own authority as an author, I have, immediately after mentioning them, carefully censored and prohibited them.

An act is never looked upon with indulgence for the simple reason that it is authorized by science, because it ought to be remembered that it is the intention of science that the rule which it contains should only be acted upon in particular cases. After reading and considering the works of Babhravya and other ancient authors, and thinking over the meaning of rules given by them, the

Kamasutra was composed according to the precepts of shastra for the benefit of the world, by Vatsyayana, while leading the life of a religious student, and wholly engaged in the contemplation of the gods.

This work is not intended to be used merely as an instrument for satisfying our desires. A person acquainted with the true principles of this science, and who preserves his Dharma, Artha and Kama, and has regard for the practices of the people is sure to obtain the mastery over his senses.

In short, an intelligent and prudent person attending to Dharma, Artha and attending to Kama also, without becoming the slave of his passions, obtains success in every thing that he may undertake.

The Arts and Sciences to be Studied

Man should study the Kamasutra and the arts and the sciences subordinate thereto in addition to the study of the arts and sciences contained in Dharma and Artha. Even young maids should study this Kamasutra along with its arts and sciences before marriage and after it they should continue to do so with the consent of their husbands. The arts that are 64 in numbers and range from making flowers, playing on musical instruments of various kinds, to knowledge of mines and quarries and warfare.

Some learned men object and say that females, not being allowed to study any science, should not study the Kamasutra. But Vatsyayana is of opinion that this objection does not hold good. If a wife becomes separated from her husband and falls into distress, she can support herself easily, even in a foreign country, by means of her knowledge of these arts. Even the bare knowledge of them gives attractiveness to a woman, although the practice of them may be only possible or otherwise according to the circumstances of each case. A man who is versed in these arts, who is loquacious and acquainted with the arts of gallantry, gains very soon the hearts of women, even though he is only acquainted with them for a short time.

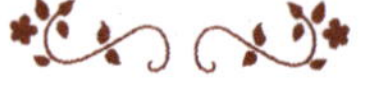

2
A Citizen's Life

Having acquired learning a man, with the wealth that he may have gained by gift, conquest, purchase, deposit or inheritance from his ancestors, should become a householder and pass the life of a citizen. He should take a house in a city, or large village or in the vicinity of good men, or in a place which is the resort of many persons. This should be situated near water and divided into compartments for different purposes. It should be surrounded by a garden, and also contain two rooms, an outer and an inner one.

The inner room should be occupied by the females, while the outer room, balmy with rich perfumes, should contain a bed, soft, agreeable to the sight covered with a clean white cloth, low in the middle part, having garlands and bunches of flowers on it and a canopy above it, and two pillows one at the top, another at the bottom. There should be also a couch besides and at the head of this stool, on which should be placed, the fragrant ointments for the night as well as flowers, pots containing collyrium and other fragrant substances, things for perfuming the mouth and the bark of the common citron tree.

Near the couch, on the ground there should be a pot for spitting, a box containing ornaments, and also a lute hanging from the peg made of the tooth of an elephant, a board for drawing, a pot containing perfume, books, and garlands of the yellow amaranth flowers, Not far from the couch and the ground there should be a round seat, a toy cart, and a board for playing with the dice; outside the outer room there should be cases of the birds and a separate place for spinning, carving and such diversions. In the garden there should be a whirling swing and a common swing, as also a bower of creepers covered with flowers in which a raised part should be made for sitting.

The householder, having got up in the morning and perform his necessary duties, should clean his teeth, apply a limited quantity of ointments and perfumes to his body, put some ornaments on his person and collyrium on his eyelids and below his eyes, colour his lips with *alaktaka* and look himself in the glass. Having then eaten betel leaves with other things that give fragrance to the mouth, he should perform his usual business. He should bathe daily, anoint his body with oil every other day, apply a lathering substance to his body every three days, get his head including his face shaved every four days and the other parts of his body every five or ten days. All these things should be done without fail, and the sweat of armpits should also be removed.

Meals should be taken in the forenoon, in the afternoon and again at night. After breakfast, parrots and other birds should be taught to speak, and the fighting of cocks, quails and rams should follow. A limited time should be devoted to diversions with Pithamardas (learned but poor men), Vitas (talkative men) and Vidushakas (clowns) and then should be taken the midday sleep. After this the householder, having put on his clothes and ornaments, should during the afternoon, converse with his friends. In the evening there should be singing, and after that the householder, along with his friend, should await in his room, decorated and perfumed, the arrival of the woman that may be attached to him, or he may send a female messenger for her, or go to her himself. After her arrival at his house, he and his friend should welcome her, and entertain with loving and agreeable conversation. Thus end the duties of the day.

The following are the things to be done occasionally as diversions or amusements.

1. *Holding festivals in honor of different deities*
2. *Social gatherings of both sexes*
3. *Drinking parties*
4. *Picnics*
5. *Other social diversions*

When kama is practised by men of four castes according to the rules of shastras, i.e. by, lawful marriage with virgins of their own castes, it then becomes a means of acquiring lawful progeny fame.

Marriage

When a girl becomes marriageable, her parents should dress her smartly and place her where she can be easily seen by all. Every afternoon, having dressed her and decorated her in a becoming manner, they should send her with her female companions to sports, sacrifices, and marriage ceremonies, and thus show her to advantage in society.

They should also receive with kind words and signs of friendliness those of an auspicious appearance who may come accompanied by their friends and relations for the purpose of marrying their daughter, and under some pretext or other, having first dressed her becomingly, should present her to them. After this they should await the pleasure of fortune, and with this object should appoint a future day on which a determination could come with regard to their daughter's marriage. On this occasion when the parents have come, the parents of the girl should ask them to bathe and dine, and say, 'Everything will take place at proper time and should not then comply with the request but should settle the matter later.

When a girl is thus acquired either according to the custom of the country, or according to his own desire, the man should marry her in accordance with the precepts of the shastras, according to one of the four kinds of marriage.

Amusement in society such as completing verses begun by others, marriage, and auspicious ceremonies should be carried on neither with superiors, nor with inferiors but with equals. That should be known as a high connection when a man, after marrying a girl, has to serve her relations afterwards like a servant, and such a connection is censured by the good. On the other hand, that reproachable connection, where a man together with his relations lords it over his wife, is called low connection by the wise. But when both the man and woman afford mutual pleasure to each other, and where the relatives on both sides pay respect to one another, such is called a connection in the proper sense of the word. Therefore, a man should contract neither a high connection by which he is obliged to bow down afterwards to his kinsmen, nor a low connection, which is universally reprehended by all.

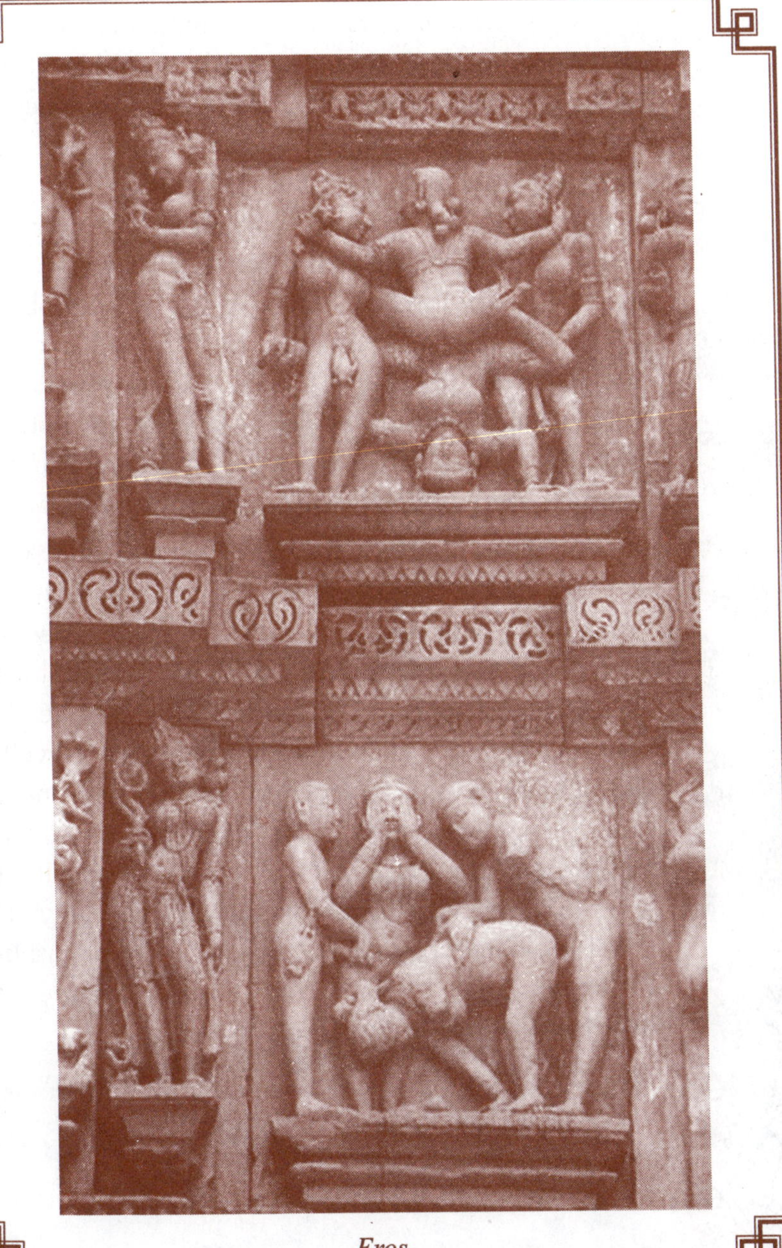

Eros

A girl who is much sought after should marry the man she likes, and whom she thinks would be obedient to her, and capable of giving her pleasure, but when from the desire of wealth a girl is married by her parents to a rich man without taking into consideration the character or looks of the bridegroom, or when given to a man who has several wives, she never becomes attached to the man, even though he be endowed with good qualities, obedient to her will, active, strong and healthy and anxious to please her in every way. **A husband who is obedient but yet master of himself, though he be poor and not good-looking, is better then one who is common to many women, even though he be handsome and attractive.**

The wives of rich men, where there are many wives, are not generally attached to their husbands, and are not confidential with them, and even though they possess all the external enjoyments of life, still have recourse to other men. A man who is of a low mind, who has fallen from his social position, and who is much given to travelling, does not deserve to be married; neither does one who has many wives and children, or one who is devoted to sport and gambling and who comes to his wife only when he likes. Of all the lovers of a girl he only is her true husband who possesses the qualities that are liked by her, and such a husband only enjoys real superiority over her, because he is the husband of love.

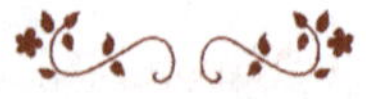

3
APPROACHING THE GIRL

For the first three days after marriage, the girl and her husband should sleep on the floor, abstain from sexual pleasures, and eat their food without seasoning it either with alkali or salt. For the next seven days they should bathe amidst the sounds of auspicious musical instruments, decorate themselves , dine together, and pay attention to their relations as well as to those who may have come to witness their marriage. This is applicable to persons of all castes. **On the night of tenth day the man should begin in a lonely place with soft words, and thus create confidence in the girl.**

Some authors say that for the purpose of winning her over he should not speak to her for three days, but the followers of Babhravya are of opinion that if the man does not speak with her for three days, the girl may be discouraged by seeing him spiritless like a pillar, and, becoming dejected, she may begin to despise him as an eunuch. Vatsyayana says that the man should begin to win her over, and to create confidence in her, but should abstain at first from sexual pleasures. Women being of a tender nature, want tender beginnings, and when they are forcibly approached by men with whom they are slightly acquainted, they sometimes suddenly become haters of sexual connection, and sometimes even haters of male sex. The man should therefore approach the girl according to her liking, and should make use of those devices by which he may be able to establish himself more and more into her confidence. These devices are as follows:

He should embrace her first of all in the way she likes most, because it does not last for a long time.

He should embrace her with the upper part of his body, because that is easier and simpler. If the girl is grown up, or if the man has known her for some time, he may embrace her by the light of a lamp, but if he is not well acquainted with her, or if she is a young girl, he should then embrace her in darkness.

When the girl accepts the embrace, the man should put a 'tambula' or piece of betel leaves and nuts in her mouth, and if she will not take it, he should induce her to do so by conciliatory words, entreaties, oaths, and kneeling at her feet, for it is a universal rule that however bashful or angry a woman may be, she never disregards a man's kneeling at her feet. At the time of giving this 'tambula' he should kiss her mouth softly and gracefully without making any sound.

When she is gained over in this way, he should then make her talk, and so that she may be induced to talk he should ask her questions about things of which he knows or pretends to know nothing, and which can be answered in a few words. If she does not speak to him, he should not frighten her, but ask the same thing again and again in a conciliatory manner. If she does not speak he should urge her to give a reply, because as Ghotakamukha says, all girls hear everything said to them by men, but do not themselves say a single word. When she is thus importuned, the girl should give replies by shakes of the head, but if she has quarrelled with the man she should not even do that. When she is asked by the man whether she wishes for him, and whether she likes him, she should remain silent for a long time, and when at last importuned to reply, she should give him a favorable answer by a nod of her head.

If the man is previously acquainted with the girl he should converse with her by means of a female friend, who may be favorable to him, and in the confidence of both, and carry on the conversation on both sides. On such an occasion the girl should smile with her head bent down, and if the female friend says more on her part than she was desired to do, she should chide her and dispute with her. The female friend should say in jest even what she is not desired to say by the girl, and add, 'she says so' on which the girl should say indistinctly and prettily. 'Oh no', 'I did not say so,' and she should then smile and throw an occasional glance towards the man.

If the girl is familiar with the man, she should place near him, without saying anything, the tambula, the ointment, or the garland that he may have asked for, or she may tie them up in his upper garment. While she is engaged in this, the man should touch her young breasts in the sounding way of pressing with the nails, and if she prevents him doing this he should say to her, 'I will not do it again if you embrace me,' and should in this way cause her to embrace him.

While he is being embraced by her, he should pass his hand repeatedly over and about her body. by and by he should place her in his lap, and try more and more to gain her consent, and if she will not yield to him he should frighten her by saying, 'I shall impress marks of my teeth and nails on your lips and breasts, and then make similar marks on my own body, and shall tell my friends that you did them. What will you say then?, In this and other ways, as fear and confidence are created

In the minds of children, so should the man gain her over to his wishes.

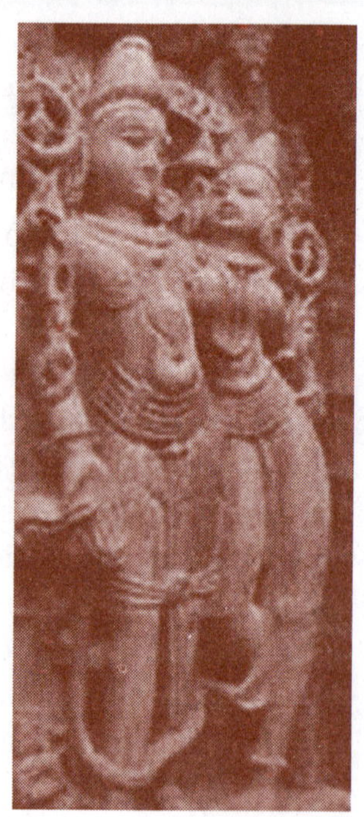

On the second and third nights, after her confidence has increased still more, he should feel the whole of her body with his hands, and kiss her all over; he should also place his hands upon her thighs and rub them, and if he succeeds in this he should then press the joints of her thighs. If she tries to prevent him doing this he should say to her, 'What harm is there in doing it?' and should then persuade her to let him do it.

After gaining this point he should touch her private parts, loosen her girdle and the knot of her dress, and turning up her lower garment should rub the joints of her naked thighs, under various pretences he should do all these things but he should not at that time begin actual, coitus. After this he shld teach her the sixty-four arts, and should tell her how much he loves her. **He should also promise to be faithful to her in future and should dispel all her fears with respect to rival women,** and, at last, after having overcome her bashfulness, he should begin to enjoy her in a way so as not to frighten her.

So much about creating confidence in the girl; and there are some verses on the subject as follows:

A man acting according to the inclinations of a girl should try and gain her over so that she may love him and place her confidence in him. A man does not succeed either by implicitly following the inclination of a girl, or by wholly opposing her, and he should therefore adopt a middle course. He who knows how to make himself beloved by women, as well as to increase their honour and create confidence in them, this man becomes the object of their love. But he, who neglects the girl thinking she is too bashful, is despised by her as a beast ignorant of the working of the female mind. Moreover, a girl forcibly enjoyed by one who does not understand the hearts of girls becomes nervous, uneasy and dejected, and suddenly begins to hate the man who has taken advantage of her; and then, when her love is not understood or returned, she sinks into despondency, and becomes either a hater of mankind altogether, or, hating her own man, she has recourse to other men.'

The Virtuous Wife

A virtuous woman, who has affection for her husband, should act in conformity with his wishes as if he were a divine being, and with his consent should take upon herself the whole care of his family. She should keep the house well cleaned, and arrange flowers of various kinds in different parts of it, and make the floor smooth and polished so as to give the whole a neat and becoming experience. She should surround the house with a garden, and place ready in it all the materials required for the morning, noon and evening sacrifices.

The wife, whether she be a woman of noble family, or a virgin widow, remarried or a concubine, should lead a chaste life, devoted to her husband and doing everything for his welfare. Women acting thus acquire Dharma, Artha and Kama, obtain a high position, and generally keep their husbands devoted to them.

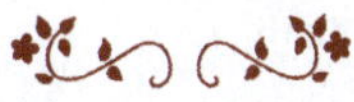

4

OTHER WOMEN

The wives of other people may be resorted to but it must be distinctly understood that it is only allowed for special reasons and not forz mere carnal desire. The possibility of their acquisition, their fitness for cohabitation, the danger to oneself in uniting with them, and the future effect of those unions, should first of all be examined. A man may resort to the wife of another, for the purpose of saving his own life, when he perceives that his love for her proceeds from one degree of intensity to another. These degrees are ten in number, and are distinguished by the following marks:

1. Love of the eye
2. Attachment of the mind
3. Constant reflection
4. Destruction of sleep
5. Emaciation of the body
6. Turning away from the objects of enjoyment
7. Removal of shame
8. Madness
9. Fainting
10. Death

The causes of a woman rejecting approaches of men are as follows:

1. Affection for her husband
2. Desire of lawful progeny
3. Want of opportunity
4. Anger of being approached by the man too familiarly
5. Difference in rank of life
6. Want of certainty on account of the man being devoted to travelling
7. Thinking that the man may be attached to some other person
8. Fear of the man not keeping his intentions secret
9. Thinking that the man is too devoted to his friends, and has too great a regard for them
10. The apprehension that he is not in earnest
11. Bashfulness on account of his being an illustrious man
12. Fear on account of his being powerful, or possessed of too impetuous passion, in the case of the 'deer' woman
13. Bashfulness on account of his being too clever
14. The thought of having once lived with him on friendly terms only
15. Contempt of his want of knowledge of the world
16. Distrust of his low character
17. Disgust at his want of her perception of her love for him
18. In the case of an 'elephant' woman, the thought that he is a 'hare' man, or a man weak of passion

19. Compassion lest anything should befall him on account of his passion
20. Despair at her own imperfections
21. Fear of discovery
22. Disillusion at seeing his grey hair or shabby appearance
23. Fear that he may be employed by her husband to test her chastity
24. The thought that he has too much regard for morality

The Harem Women

The women of the royal harem cannot see or meet any men on account of their being strictly guarded, neither do they give pleasure to each other in various ways as now described.

Having dressed the daughters of their nurses, or their female friends, or their female attendants like men, they accomplished their objects by means of bulbs, roots, and fruits having the form of penis, or they lie down upon the statue of a male figure, in which the penis is visible and erect.

Some kings, who are compassionate, take or apply certain medicines to enable them to enjoy many wives in one night, simply for the purpose of satisfying the desire of their women, though they perhaps have no desire of their own. Others enjoy with great affection only those wives that they particularly like, while others only take them, according as the turn of each wife arrives, in due course.

By means of their female attendants the ladies of the royal harem generally get men into their apartments in the disguise or dress of women. Their female attendants and the daughters of their nurses, who are acquainted with their secrets, should exert themselves to get men to come to the harem in this way by telling them of the good fortune attending it, and by describing the facilities of entering and leaving the palace, the large size of the premises, the carelessness of the sentinels, and the irregularities of the attendants about the persons of royal wives. But these women should never induce a man to enter the harem by telling him falsehoods, for that would probably lead to his destruction.

The entrance of young men into harems, and their exits from them, generally take place when things are being brought into the palace, or when the things are being taken out of it, or when drinking festivals are going on, or when female attendants are in a hurry, or when the residence of some of the royal ladies is being changed, or when the king's wives go to the gardens, or to fairs, or when they enter the palace on their return from them, or, lastly, when the king is absent on a long pilgrimage. The women of the royal harem know each other's secrets, and having but one object to attain, they give assistance to each other. A young man, who enjoys all of them, and who is common to them all, can continue enjoying his union with them so long as it is kept quiet, and is not known abroad.

Thus act the wives of others.

For these reasons a man should guard his own wife.

The followers of Babhravya say that a man should cause his wife to associate with a young man who would tell him the secrets of other people, and thus find out from her about his wife's chastity. But Vatsyayana says that as the wicked persons are always successful with women, a man should not cause his innocent wife to be corrupted by bringing her into the company of a deceitful woman.

The following are the causes of the destruction of a woman's chastity:

- Always going into society, and sitting in company
- Absence of restraint
- The loose habits of her husband
- Want of caution in her relations with other men
- Continued and long absence of her husband
- Living in a foreign country
- Destruction of her love and feelings by her husband
- The company of loose women
- The jealousy of her husband

There are also the following verses on the subject:

'*A clever man, learning from Shastras the way of winning over the wives of other people, is never deceived in the case of his own wives. No-one, however, should make of these ways for seducing the wives of others, because they do not always succeed, and moreover, often cause disasters, and the destruction of Dharma and Artha. This book, which is intended for the good of the people, and to teach them the ways of guarding their own wives, should not be made use of merely for gaining over the wives of others.*'

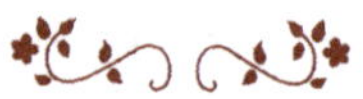

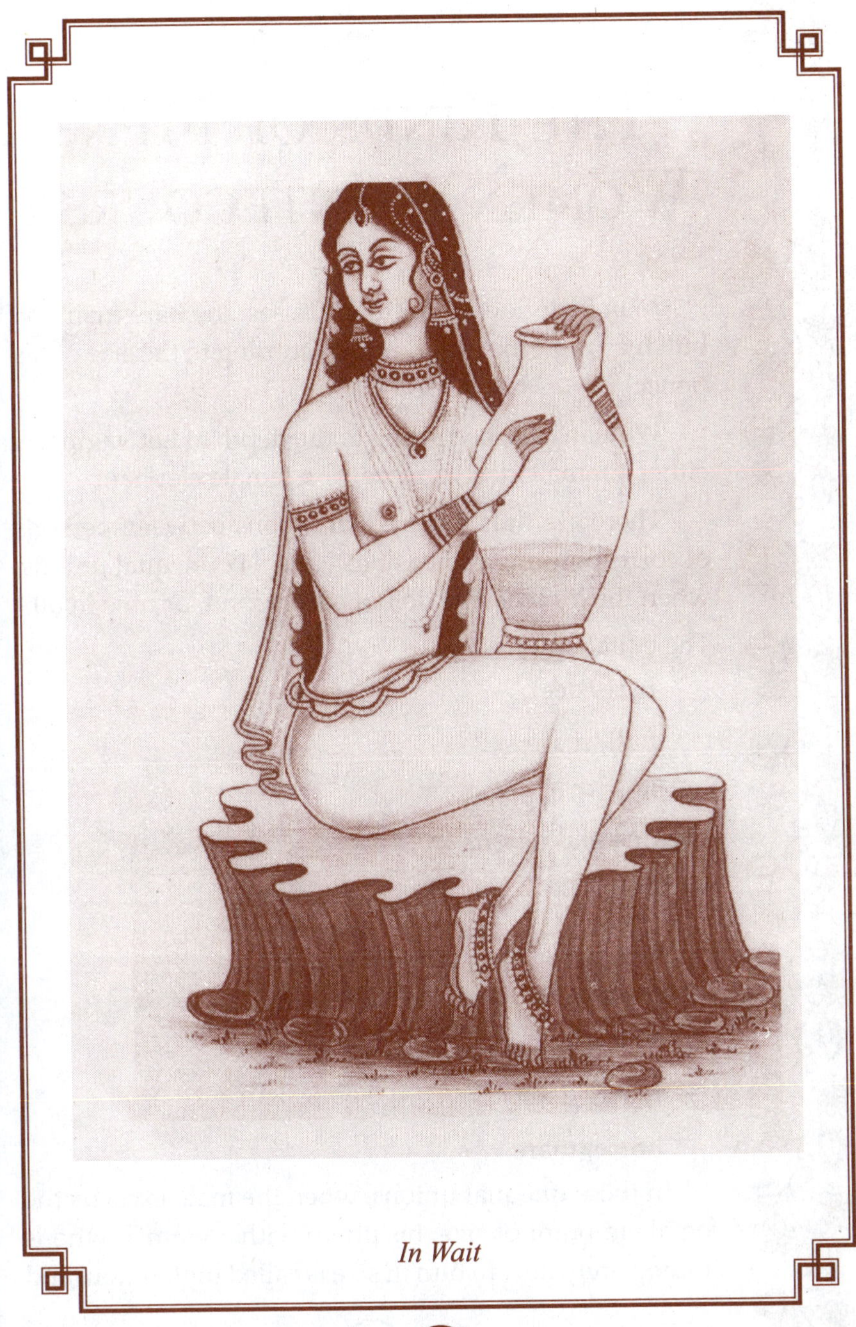

In Wait

5
The Kinds of Men, Women & Intecourse

Man is divided into three classes: the hare man, the bull man, and the horse man, according to the size of his penis.

Woman also, according to the depth of her vagina, is either a female deer, a mare, or a female elephant.

There are thus three equal unions between persons of corresponding dimensions, and six unequal unions, when the dimensions do not correspond, or nine in all. The equal unions are:

hare/deer;

bull/mare;

horse/elephant.

The unequal unions are:

hare/mare;

hare/elephant;

bull/deer;

bull/elephant;

horse/deer;

horse/mare.

In these unequal unions, when the male exceeds the female in point of size, his union with a woman who is immediately next to him in size is called high union, and is of two kinds; while his union with the woman most remote from him in size is called the highest union, and is of one kind only. On the other hand, when the female exceeds the male in point of size, her union with a man immediately next to her in size is called low union, and is of two kinds; while her union with a man most remote from her in size is called the lowest union, and is of one kind only.

In other words, the horse and mare, the bull and deer, form the high union, while the horse and deer form the highest union. On the female side, the elephant and bull, the mare and hare, form low unions, while the elephant and the hare make the lowest union.

The Nine Kinds of Union

There are then, nine kinds of union according to dimensions. Among all these, equal unions are the best, those of a superlative degree, i.e., the highest and the lowest are the worst, and the rest are middling, and with them the high are better than the low.

There are also nine kinds of union according to the force of passion or carnal desire. The three equal unions are when both partners have either small, middling or intense passion. The unequal unions are small/ middling/ small; and intense/ middling/ small middling.

A man is called a man of small passion whose desire at the time of sexual union is not great, whose semen is scanty, and who cannot bear the warm embraces of the female.

Those who differ from this temperament are called men of middling passion, while those of intense passion are full of desire.

In the same way, women are supposed to have the three degrees of feeling as specified above.

Lastly, according to time there are three kinds of men and women: the short-timed, the moderate-timed and the long-timed, and of these as in the previous statements, there are nine kinds of union.

Do Women Eject?

But on this last head there is a difference of opinion about the female, which should be stated.

Auddalaka, an authority on the subject:, says. 'Females do not eject as males do. The males simply remove their pleasure, which gives them satisfaction, but it is impossible for them to tell you what kind of pleasure they feel. The fact from which this becomes evident is, that males, when engaged in coition, cease of themselves after ejection, and are satisfied, but it is not so with females.'

This opinion is however objected to on the grounds that if male be long-timed, the female loves him the more, but if he be short-timed, she is dissatisfied with him and this circumstance, some would say, would prove that the female also ejects.

But this opinion does not hold good, for if it takes a long time to allay a woman's desire, and during this time she is enjoying great pleasure, it is quite natural that she should wish for its continuation, and on this subject there is a verse as follows:

'By union with men the lust, desire, or passion of women is satisfied, and the pleasure derived from the consciousness of it is called their satisfaction.'

The followers of Babhravya, however, say that the semen of women continues to fall from the beginning of the sexual union to its end, and it is right that it should be so, for if they had no semen there would be no embryo.

To this there is an objection, In the beginning of coition the passion of the woman is middling, and she cannot bear the vigorous thrust of her lover, but by degrees her passion increases until she ceases to think about her body, and then finally she wishes to stop from further coition.

This objection, however, does not hold good, for even in ordinary things that revolve with great force, such as potter's wheel, or a top, we find that the motion at first is slow, but by degrees it becomes very rapid. In the same way, the passion of the woman having gradually increased she has a desire to discontinue coition, when all the semen has fallen away. And there is a verse with regard to this as follows:

'*The fall of the semen of the man takes place only at the end of coition, while the semen of the woman falls continually, and after the semen of both has all fallen away, they wish for the discontinuance of coition.*'

Lastly, Vatsyayana is of opinion that the semen of the female falls in the same way as that of the male.

Someone may ask if men and women are beings of the same kind, and are engaged in bringing about the same result, why should they have different acts to do.

Vatsyayana says that this is so because the ways of acting as well as the consciouness of pleasure in men and women are different. The difference in the ways of acting by which men are the actors, and women are the persons acted upon, is owing to the nature of the male and the female, otherwise the actor would be sometimes the person acted upon, and vice versa. And from this difference in the ways of acting follows the difference in the consciousness of pleasure, for a man thinks, this woman is united with me, and a woman thinks, I am united with the man.

It may be said that if the ways of men and women are different, why should not there be a difference, even in the pleasure they feel, and which is the result of those ways.

But this objection is groundless, for the person acting and the person acted upon being of different kinds, there is a reason for the difference in their way of acting but there is no reason for any difference in the pleasure they feel, because they both naturally derive pleasure from the act they perform.

On this again some may say that when different persons are engaged in doing the same act, we find that they accomplish the same end or purpose; while, on the contrary, in the case of men and women we find that each of them accomplished his or her own separately, and this in inconsistent. But this is a mistake, for we find that sometimes two things are done at the same time, as for instance in the fighting of rams, both the rams receive the shock at the same time on their heads, Again, in throwing one wood apple against another, and also in a fight or struggle of wrestlers, if it be said that in these cases the things employed are of the same kind, it is answered that even in the case of men and women, the nature of the two persons is the same. And as the difference is of their conformation only, it follows that men experience the same kind of pleasure as women do.

There is also a verse on this subject as follows:

'Men and women being of the same nature, feel the same kind of pleasure, and therefore a man should marry such a woman as will love him ever afterwards.'

The pleasure of men and women being thus proved to be of the same kind, it follows that in regard to time, there are nine kinds of sexual intercourse, in the same way as there are nine kinds according to the force of passion.

There being thus nine kinds of union with regard to dimensions, force of passion, and time, respectively, by making combinations of them, innumerable kinds of union would be produced. Therefore in each particular kind of sexual union, men should use such means as they may think suitable for the occasion.

At the first time of sexual union the passion of the man is intense, and his time is short, but in subsequent unions on the same day the reverse of this is the case. With the female however it is the contrary, for at the first time her passion is weak, and then her time long, but on subsequent occasions on the same day, her passion is intense and her time short, until her passion is satisfied.

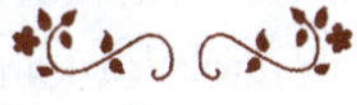

6
Love-making

Men learned in the humanities are of opinion that love is of four kinds:

1. Love acquired by continual habit
2. Love resulting from the imagination
3. Love resulting from belief
4. Love resulting from the perception of external objects

1) Love resulting from the constant and continual performance of some act is called love acquired by constant practice and habit, as for instance, the love of sexual intercourse, the love of hunting, the love of drinking, the love of gambling, etc.

2) Love which is felt for things to which we are not habituated, and which proceeds entirely from ideas, is called love resulting from imagination, as for instance, that love which some men and women and eunuchs feel for the Auparishtaka or mouth-congress, and that which is felt by all for such things as embracing, kissing, etc.

3) The love which is mutual on both sides, and proved to be true, when each looks upon the other as his or her very own, such is called love resulting from belief, by the learned.

4) The love resulting from the perception of external objects is quite evident and well-known to the world,

because the pleasure which it affords is superior to the pleasure of the other kinds of love, which exist for its sake.

What has been said in this chapter upon the subject of sexual union is sufficient for the learned; but for the edification of the ignorant, the same will now be treated of at length and in detail.

The Embrace

This part of the Kama Shastra, which treats of sexual union, is also called 'Sixty-four' (Chatushshashti). Some old authors say that it is called so, because it contains sixty-four chapters. The followers of Babhravya say on the other hand that this part contains eight subjects: the embrace, kissing, scratching with the nails or fingers, biting, lying down, making various sounds, playing the part of a man, and the Auparishtaka, or mouth-congress. Each of these subjects being of eight kinds, and eight multiplied by eight being sixty-four, this part is therefore named 'Sixty-four'. But Vatsyayana affirms that as this part contains also the following subjects: striking, crying, the acts of a man during the various kinds of coition and other subjects, the name 'Sixty-four' is given to it only accidentally.

However, the part is now treated of, and the embrace, being the first subject, will now be considered.

The embrace which indicates the mutual love of a man and woman who have come together is of four kinds:

Touching	Rubbing
Piercing	Pressing

The action in each case is denoted by the meaning of the word which stands for it.

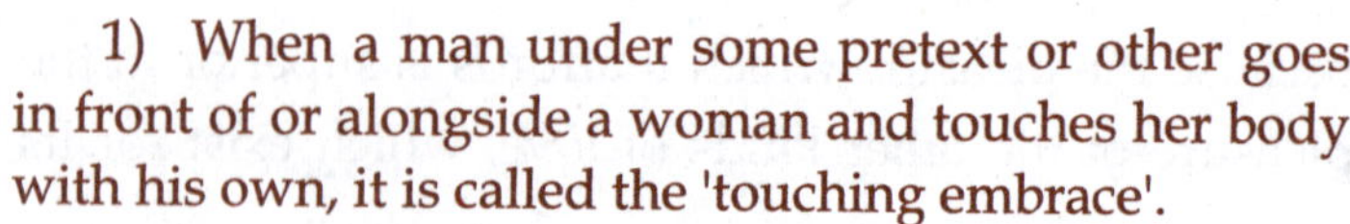

1) When a man under some pretext or other goes in front of or alongside a woman and touches her body with his own, it is called the 'touching embrace'.

2) When a woman in a lonely place bends down, as if to pick up something, and pierces, as it were, a man sitting or standing, with her breasts, and the man in return takes hold of them, it is called a 'piercing embrace'.

The above two kinds of embrace take place only between persons who do not, as yet, speak freely with each other.

3) When two lovers are walking slowly together, either in the dark, or in a place of public resort, or in a lonely place, and rub their bodies against each other, it is called a 'rubbing embrace'.

4) When on the above occasion one of them presses the other's body forcibly against a wall or pillar, it is called a 'pressing embrace'.

These last two embraces are peculiar to those who know the intentions of each other.

At the time of meetings the four following kinds of embrace are used:

Jataveshtitaka, or the twining of a creeper

Vrikshadhirudhaka, or climbing a tree

Tila-tandulaka, or the mixture of sesamum seed with rice

Kshiraniraka, or milk and water embrace

1) When a woman, clinging to a man as a creeper twines round a tree, bends his head down to hers with the desire of kissing him and slightly makes the sound of *sut sut*, embraces him, and looks lovingly towards him, it is called an embrace like the 'twining of a creeper'.

2) When a woman, having placed one of her feet on the foot of her lover, and the other on one of his thighs, passes one of her arms round his back, and the other on his shoulders, makes slightly the sounds of singing and cooing, and wishes, as it were, to climb up to him in order to have a kiss, it is called an embrace like the 'climbing of a tree'.

These two kinds of embrace take place when the lover is standing.

3) When lovers lie on a bed, and embrace each other so closely that the arms and thighs of the one are encircled by the arms and thighs of the other, and are, as it were, rubbing up against them, this is called an embrace like the 'mixture of sesamum seed with rice.'

4) When a man and a woman are very much in love with each other and, not thinking of any pain or hurt, embrace each other as if they were entering into each other's bodies either while the woman is sitting on the lap of the man, or in front of him, or on a bed, then it is called an embrace like a 'mixture of milk and water'.

These two kinds of embrace take place at the time of sexual union.

Babhravya has thus related to us the above eight kinds of embraces.

Suvarnanabha moreover gives us four ways of embracing simple members of the body, which are:

The embrace of the thighs

The embrace of the *jaghana*, the part of the body from the navel downwards to the thighs

The embrace of the breasts

The embrace of the forehead

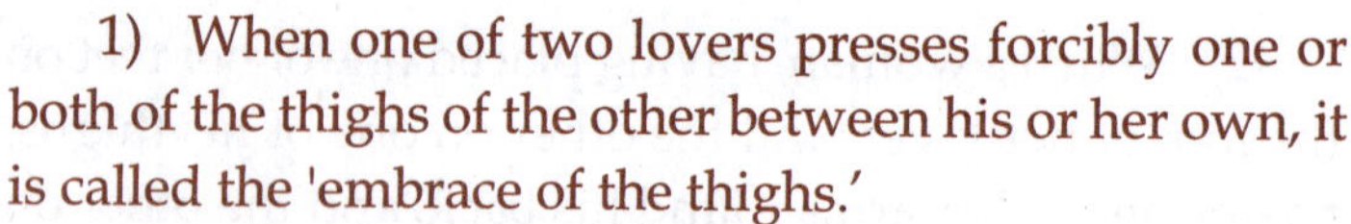

1) When one of two lovers presses forcibly one or both of the thighs of the other between his or her own, it is called the 'embrace of the thighs.'

2) When the man presses the *jaghana* or middle part of the woman's body against his own, and mounts upon her to practise either scratching with the nail or finger, or biting, or striking, or kissing, the hair of the woman being loose and flowing, it is called the, embrace of the *jaghana*'.

3) When a man places his breast between the breasts of a woman and presses her with it, it is called the 'embrace of the breasts'.

4) When either of the lovers touches the mouth, the eyes and the forehead of the other with his or her own, it is called the 'embrace of the forehead.

Some say that even rubbing is a kind of embrace, because there is a touching of bodies in it. But Vatsyayana thinks that rubbing is performed at a different time, and for a different purpose, and as it is also of a different character, it cannot be said to be included in the embrace.

There are also some verses on the subject as follows:

'*The whole subject of embracing is of such a nature that men who ask questions about it, or who hear about it, or who talk about it, acquire thereby a desire for enjoyment. Even those embraces that are not mentioned in the Kama Shastra should be practiced at the time of sexual enjoyment, if they are in any way conducive to the increase of love or passion. The rules of the Shastra apply so long as the passion of man is middling, but when the wheel of love is once set in motion, there is then no Shastra and no order.*

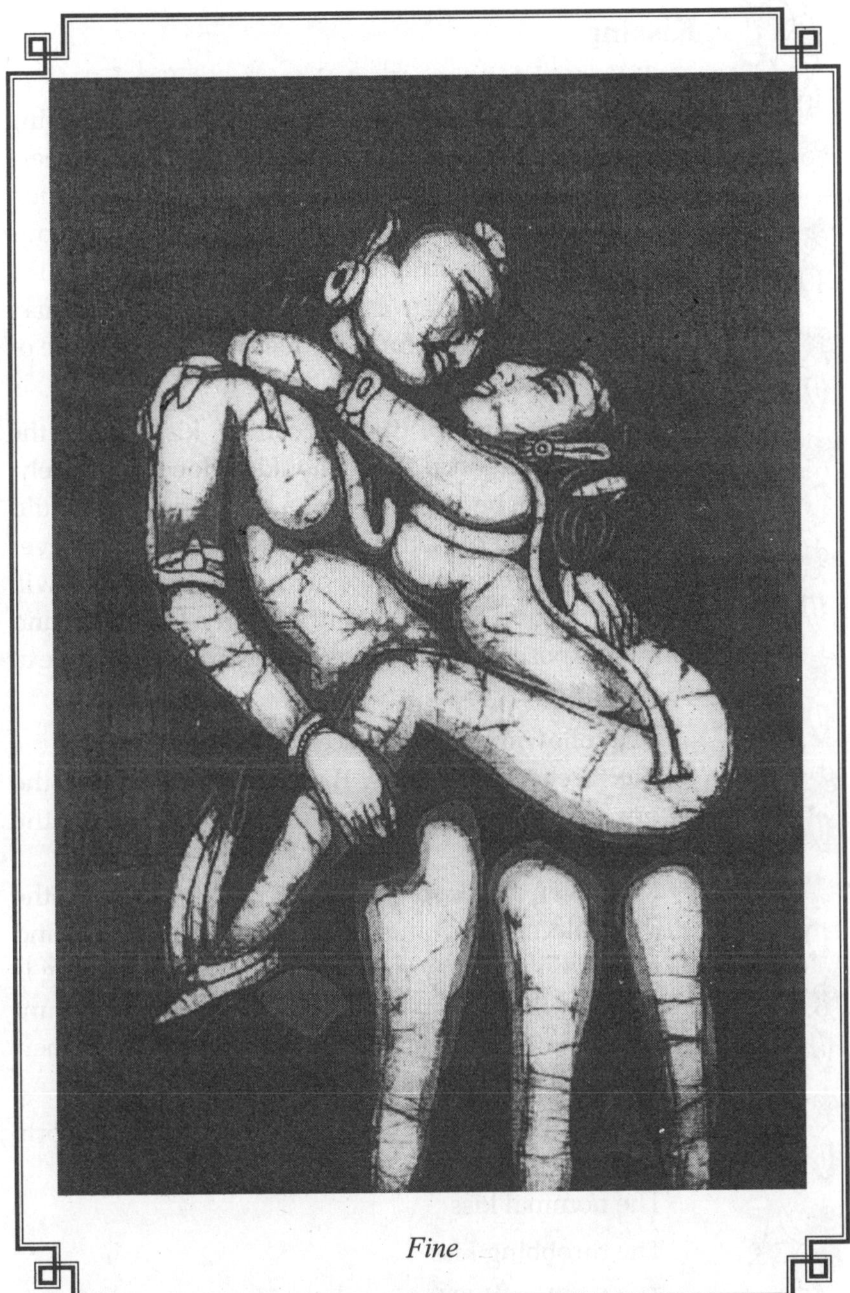

Fine

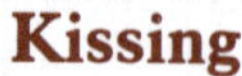

Kissing

It is said by some that there is no fixed time or order between the embrace, the kiss, and the pressing or scratching with the nails or fingers, but that all there things should be done generally before sexual union takes place, while striking and making the various moves should generally take place at the time of the union. Vatsyayana, however, thinks that anything may take place at any time, for love does not care for time or order.

On the occasion of the first coition, kissing and the other things mentioned above should be done moderately, they should not be continued for a long time, and should be done alternately. On subsequent occasions however the reverse of all this may take place, and moderation will not be necessary; they may continue for a long time, and for the purpose of kindling love, they may all be done at the same time.

The following are the places for kissing:

the forehead, the eyes, the cheeks, the throat, the bosom, the breasts, the lips and the interior of the mouth.

Moreover, the people of the Lat country kiss also the follwing places: the joints of the thighs, the arms, and the navel. But Vatsyayana thinks that though kissing is practised by these people in the above places on account of the intensity of their love, and the customs of their country, it is not fit to be practised by all.

Now in the case of a young girl there are three sorts of kisses:

The nominal kiss

The throbbing kiss

The touching kiss

1) When a girl only touches the mouth of her lover with her own, but does not herself do anyhing, it is called 'the nominal kiss.'

2) When a girl, setting aside her bashfulness a little, wishes to touch the lip that is pressed into her mouth, and with that object moves her lower, lip, but not the upper one, it is called the 'throbbing kiss'.

3) When a girl touches her lovers' lip with her tongue, and having shut her eyes, places her hands on those of her lover, it is called the 'touching kiss.'

Other authors describe four other kinds of kisses:

The straight kiss

The bent kiss

The turned kiss

The pressed kiss

1) When the lips of two lovers are brought into direct contact with each other, it is called a 'straight kiss'.

2) When the heads of two lovers are bent towards each other, and when so bent, kissing takes place, it is called a 'bent kiss.'

3) When one of them turns up the face of the other by holding the head and chin, and then kissing, it is called a 'turned kiss.'

4) Lastly, when the lower lip is pressed with much force, it is called a 'pressed kiss.'

There is also a fifth kind of kiss called the 'greatly pressed kiss', which is effected by taking hold of the lower lip between two fingers, and then after touching it with the tongue, pressing it with great force with the lip.

As regards kissing, a wager may be laid as to which will get hold of the lips of the other first, if the women loses, she should pretend to cry, should keep her lover off by shaking her hands, and turn away from him and dispute with him saying 'let another wager be laid'.

If she loses this a second time, she should appear doubly distressed, and when her lover is off his guard or asleep, she should get hold of his lower lip, and hold it in her teeth, so that it should not slip away, and then she should laugh, make a loud noise, deride him, dance about, and say whatever she likes in a joking way, moving her eyebrows, and rolling her eyes. Such are the wagers and quarrels as far as kissing is concerned, but the same may be applied with regard to the pressing or scratching with the nails and fingers, biting and striking. All these however are only peculiar to men and women of intense passion.

When a man kisses the upper lip of a woman, while she in return kisses his lower lip, it is called the 'kiss of the upper lip'.

When one of them takes both the lips of the other between his or her own, it is called a 'clasping kiss'. A woman, however, only takes this kind of kiss from a man with no moustache. And on the occasion of this kiss, if one of them touches the teeth, the tongue, and the palate of the other, with his or her tongue, it is called the 'fighting of the tongue.' In the same way, the pressing of the teeth of the one against the mouth of the other is to be practiced.

Kissing is of four kinds: moderate, contracted, pressed, and soft, according to the different parts of the body which are kissed, for different kinds of kisses are appropriate for different parts of the body.

When a woman looks at the face of her lover while

he is asleep, and kisses it to show her intention or desire, it is called a 'kiss that kindles love'.

When a woman kisses her lover while he is engaged in business, or he is quarrelling with her, or while he is looking at something else, so that his mind may be turned away, it is called a 'kiss that turns away.'

When a lover coming home late at night kisses his beloved who is asleep on her bed in order to show her his desire, it is called a 'kiss that awakens'. On such an occasion the woman may pretend to be asleep at the time of her lover's arrival, so that she may know his intention and obtain respect from him.

When a persons kisses the reflection of the person he loves in a mirror, in water, or on a wall, it is called a 'kiss showing the inteintion'.

When a person kisses a child sitting on his lap, or a picture, or an image or figure, in the presence of the person beloved by him, it is called a 'transferred kiss'.

When at night at a theatre, or in an assembly of caste men, a man coming up to a woman kisses a finger of her hand if she be standing, or a toe of her foot if she be sitting, or when a woman in rubbing her lover's body, places her face on his thigh (as if she was sleepy) so as to inflame his passion, and kisses his thigh or great toe, it is called a 'demonstrative kiss.'

There is also a verse on this subject as follows:

'Whatever things may be done by one of the lovers to the other, if the woman kisses him he should kiss her in return, if she strikes him he should also strike her in return.'

Pressing, Marking, Scratching

When love becomes intense, pressing with the nails or scratching the body with them is practiced, and it is done on the following occasions: on the first visit; at the time of setting out on a journey; on the return from a journey; at the time when any angry lover is reconciled; and lastly, when the woman is intoxicated.

But pressing with the nails is not a usual thing except with those who are intensely passionate. It is employed together with biting, by those to whom the practice is agreeable. Pressing with the nails is of the eight following kinds, according to the forms of the marks which are produced:

1. Sounding
2. Half moon
3. A circle
4. A line
5. A tiger's nail or claw
6. A peacock's foot
7. The jump of a hare
8. The leaf of a blue lotus.

The places that are to be pressed with the nails are as follows;

The armpit, the throat, the breasts, the lips, the *jaghana* or middle parts of the body, and the thighs. But Suvarnanabha is of the opinion that when the impetuosity of passion is excessive, then the places need not be considered.

The qualities of good nails are that they should be bright, well set, clean, entire, convex, soft and glossy in appearance. Nails are of three kinds according to their size:

Small Middling Large

Small nails, which can be used in various ways, and

are to be applied only with the object of giving pleasure, are possessed by the people of the southern districts.

Large nails, which give grace to the hands, and attract the hearts of women from their appearance, are possessed by the Bengalis.

Middling nails, which contain the properties of both the above kinds, belong to the people of Maharashtra.

1) When a person presses the chin, the breasts, the lower lip or the *jaghana* of another so softly that no scratch or mark is left, but only the hair on the body become erect from the touch of the nails, and the nails themselves make a sound, it is called 'sounding or pressing with the nails'. This pressing is used in the case of a young girl when her lover rubs her, scratches her head, and wants to trouble or frighten her.

2) The curved mark with the nails, which is impressed on the neck and the breasts is called the 'half moon.'

3) When the half moons are impressed opposite to each other, it is called circle. This mark with the nails is generally made on the navel, the small cavities about the buttocks, and on the joints of the thigh.

4) A mark in the form of a small line, and which can be made on any part of the body, is called a 'line'.

5) This same line, when it is curved, and made on the breast, is called a 'tiger's nail.'

6) When a curved mark is made on the breast by means of the five nails, it is called 'peacock's foot'. This mark is made with the object of being praised, for it requires a great deal of skill to make it properly.

7) When five marks with the nails are made close to one another near the nipple of the breast, it is called the 'jump of a hare'.

8) A mark made on the breast or on the hips in the form of a leaf of the blue lotus, is called the 'leaf of a blue lotus.'

When a person is going on a long journey, and makes a mark on the thighs, or on the breast, it is called a 'token of remembrance'. On such an occasion three or four lines are impressed close to one another with the nails.

Here ends the marking with the nails. Marks of other kinds than the above may also be made with the nails, for the ancient authors say, that as there are innumerable degrees of skill among men (the practice of this art being known, to all), so there are innumerable ways of making these marks. And as pressing or marking with the nails is dependent on love, no one can say with certainty how many different kinds of marks with the nails do actually exist. The reason of this is, Vatsyayana says, **that as variety is necessary in love, so love is to be produced by means of variety.** It is on this account that courtesans, who are well acquainted with the various ways and means, become so desirable, for if variety is sought in all the arts and amusements, such as archery and others, how much more should it be sought after in the present case.

The marks of the nails should not be made on married women, but particular kinds of marks may be made on their private parts for the remembrance and increase of love.

There are also some verses on the subject, as follows:

'The love of a woman who sees the marks of nails on the private parts of her body, even though they are old and almost worn out, becomes again fresh and new, if there be no marks

of nails to remind a person of the passages of love, then love lessened in the same way as when no union takes place for a long time.'

Even when a stranger sees at a distance a young woman with the marks of nails on her breasts he is filled with love and respect for her.

A man, also, who carries the marks of nails and teeth on some parts of his body, influences the mind of a woman, even though it be ever so firm. In short, nothing tends to increase love so much as the effects of marking with the nails, and biting.

Biting

All the places that can be kissed, are also the places that can be bitten, except the upper lip, the interior of the mouth, and the eyes.

The qualities of good teeth are as follows:

They should be equal, possessed of a pleasing brightness, capable of being coloured, of proper proportions, unbroken, and with sharp ends.

The defects of teeth on the other hand are:

They are blunt, protruding from the gums, rough, soft, large and loosely set.

The following are the different kinds of biting:

The hidden bite

The swollen bite

The point

The line of points

The coral and the jewel

The line of jewels

The broken cloud

The biting of the boar

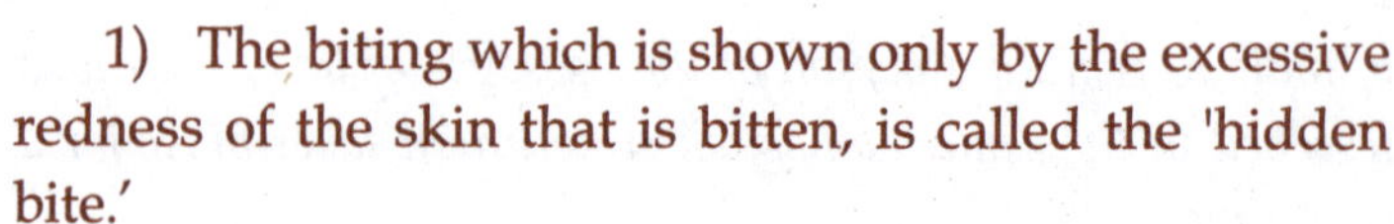

1) The biting which is shown only by the excessive redness of the skin that is bitten, is called the 'hidden bite.'

2) When the skin is pressed down on both sides, it is called the 'swollen bite'.

3) When a small portion of the skin is bitten with two teeth only, it is called the 'point'.

4) When such small portions of the skin are bitten with all the teeth, it is called the 'line of points'.

5) The biting which is done by bringing together the teeth and the lips, is called the 'coral and the jewel'. The lip is the coral, and the teeth the jewel.

6) When the biting is done with all the teeth, it is called the 'line of jewels'.

7) The biting which consists of unequal risings in a circle and which comes form the space between the teeth, is called the 'broken cloud'. This is impressed on the breasts.

8) The biting which consists of many broad rows of marks near to one another, and with red internals, is called 'the biting of a boar'. This is impressed on the breasts and the shoulders; and these two last modes of biting are peculiar to persons of intense passion.

The lower lip is the place on which the hidden bite, the swollen bite, and the point are made; again the swollen bite, and the coral, the jewel bite are done on the cheek. Kissing, pressing with the nails, and biting are the ornaments of the left cheek, and when the word cheek is used, it is to be understood as the left cheek.

Both the line of points and the line of jewels are to be impressed on the throat, the armpit and the joints of the thighs; but the line of points along is to be impressed on the forehead and the thighs.

The marking with the nails, and the biting of the following things: an ornament of the forehead, an ear ornament, a bunch of flowers, a betel leaf, or a *tamala* leaf, which are worn by, or belong to the woman that is beloved, are signs of the desire of enjoyment.

Among the things mentioned above, embracing, kissing, etc., those which increase passion should be done first, and those which are only for amusement or variety should be done afterwards.

There are also some verses on this subject as follows:

'When a man bites a woman forcibly, she should angrily do the same to him with double force. Thus a point should be returned with a line of points, and a line of points with a broken cloud, and if she be excessively chafed, she should at once begin a love quarrel with him. At such time she should take hold of her lover by the hair, and bend his head down, and kiss his lower lip, and then, being intoxicated with love, she should shut her eyes and bite him in various places. Even by day, and in a place of public resort, when her lover shows her any mark that she may have inflicted on his body, she should smile at the sight of it, and turning her face as if she were going to chide him, she should show him with an angry look the marks on her own body that have been made by him. Thus if men and women act according to each other's liking, their love for each other will not be lessened even in one hundred years.'

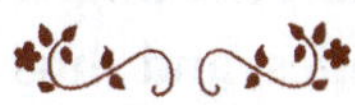

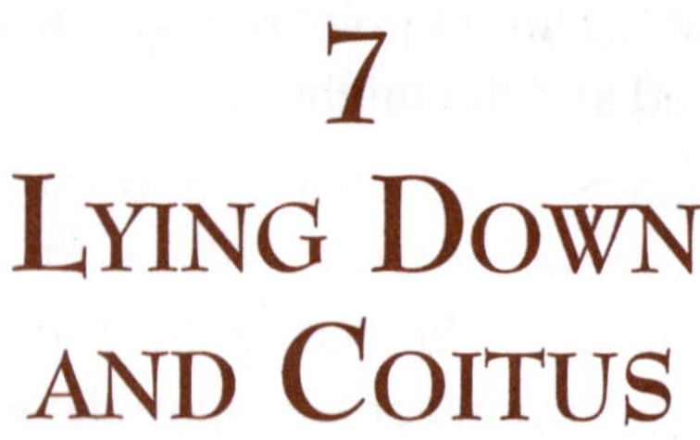

7
Lying Down and Coitus

On the occasion of a high congress the deer woman should lie down in such a way as to widen her vagina, while in a low congress the elephant woman should lie down so as to contract hers. But in an equal congress they should lie down in the natural position. What is said above concerning the deer/elephant applies also to the mare woman. In a low congress the women should particularly make use of medicine, to cause her desires to be satisfied quickly.

The deer woman has the following three ways of lying down:

The widely opened position

The yawning position

The position of the wife of Indra

1) When she lowers her head and raises her middle parts, it is called the 'widely' opened position, At such time the man should apply some unguent, so as to make the entrance easy.

2) When she raises her thighs and keeps them wide apart and engages in congress, it is called the 'yawning postion'.

3) When she places her thighs with her legs doubled on them upon her sides, and thus engages in congress, it is called the 'position of Indrani' and this is learnt only by practice. The postion is also useful in the case of the

highest congress, together with the pressing position, the twining position and the mare's position.

When the legs of both the male and the female are stretched straight out over each other, it is called the 'clasping position'. It is of two kinds, the side position and the supine postion, according to the way in which they lie down. In the side position the male should invariably lie on his left side, and cause the woman to lie on her right side, and this rule is to be observed in lying down with all kinds of women.

When, after congress has begun in the clasping position, the woman presses her lover with her thighs , it is called the 'pressing position'.

When the woman places one of her thighs across the thigh of her lover, it is c alled the 'twining position'.

When the woman forcibly holds in her vagina the penis after it is in, it is called the 'mare's position'. This is learnt by practice only, and is chiefly found among the women of the Andhra country.

The above are the different ways of lying down, mentioned by Babhravya. Suvarnanabha, however, gives the following in addtion:

When the female raises both of her thighs straight up, it is called 'the rising position'.

When she raises both of her legs, and places them on her lover's shoulders, it is called 'the vyawning the position'.

When the legs are contracted, and thus held by the lover before his bosom, it is called 'the pressed position'.

When only one of her legs is stretched out, it is called

'the half pressed position'.

When the woman places one of her legs on her lover's shoulder and stretches the other out, then places the latter on his shoulder, and stretches out the other, and continues to do so alternately, it is called the 'splitting of a bamboo'.

When one of her legs is placed on the head, and the other is stretched out, it is called the 'fixing of a nail'. This is learnt by practice only.

When both the legs of the woman are contracted, and placed on her stomach, it is called the 'crab's position'.

When the thighs are raised and placed on upon the other, it is called the 'packed position'.

When the shanks are placed one upon the other, it is called 'the lotus-like position'.

When a man, during congress, turns round, and enjoys the woman without leaving her, while she embraces him round the back all the time, it is called the 'turning position', and is learnt only by practice.

Thus, says Suvarnanabha, these different ways of lying down, sitting, and standing should be practised in water, because it is easy to do therein. But Vatsyayana is of the opinion that congress in water is improper, because it is prohibited by the religious law.

When a man and a woman support themselves on each other's bodies, or on a wall, or pillar, and thus while standing engage in congress, it is called the 'supported congress'.

When a man supports himself against a wall, and the woman, sitting on his hand joined together and held

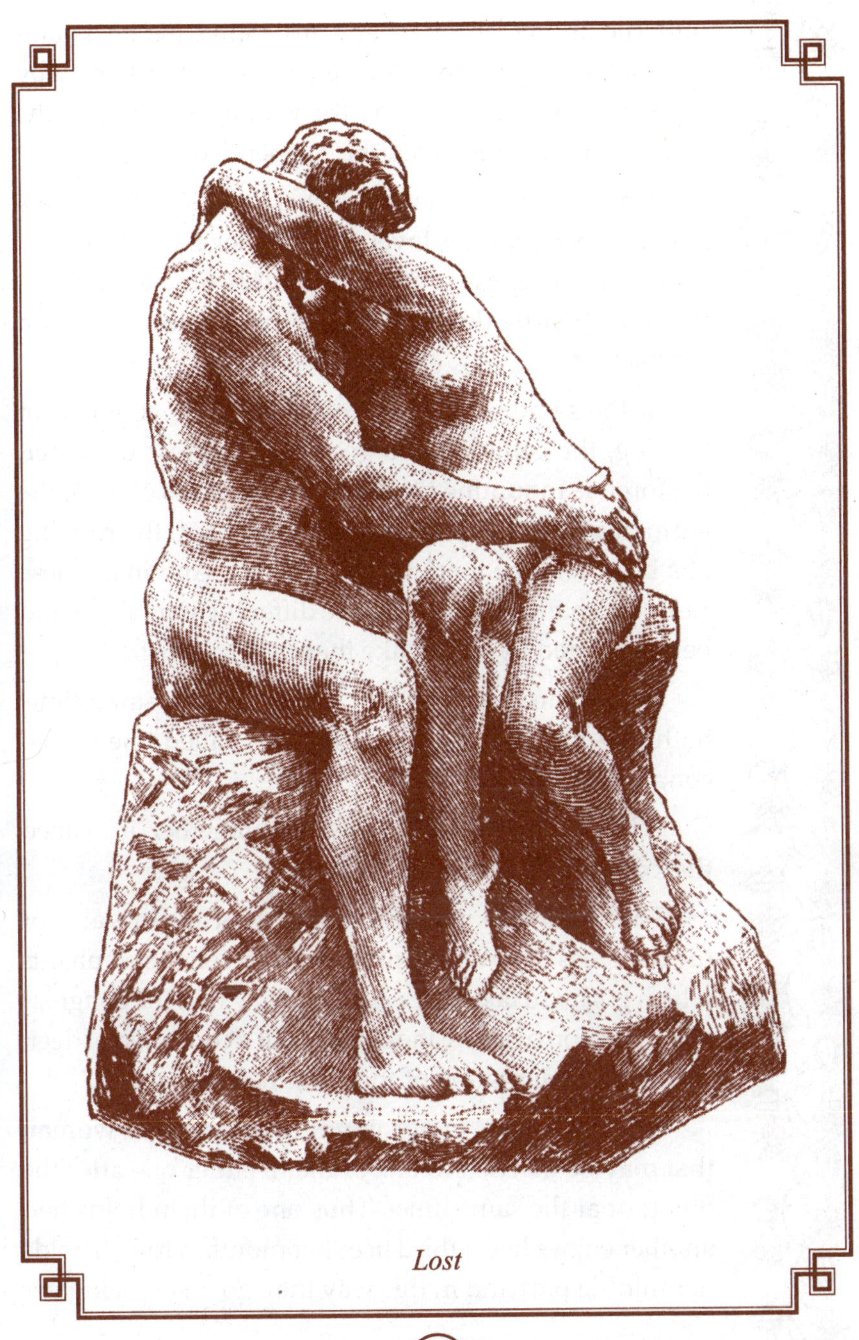

Lost

underneath her, throws her arms round his neck, and putting her thighs alongside his waist, moves herself by her feet which are touching the wall against which the man is leaning, it is called the 'suspended congress'.

When a woman stands on her hands and feet like a quadruped and her lover mounts her like a bull, it is called the 'congress of a cow'. At this time everything that is ordinarily done on the bosom should be done on the back.

In the same way can be carried on the congress of the dog, the congress of a goat, the congress of a deer, the forcible mounting of an ass, the congress of a cat, the jump of a tiger, the pressing of an elephant, the rubbing of a boar, and the mounting of a horse. And in all these cases the characteristics of these different animals should be manifested by acting like them.

When a man enjoys two women at the same time, both of whom love him equally, it is called 'the united congress'.

When a man enjoys many women together, it is called the 'congress of a herd of cows'.

The following kinds of congress: sporting in water, or the congress of an elephant with many female elephants which is said to take place only in the water, the congress of a collection of goats, the congress of a collection of deer, take place in imitation of these animals.

In Gramaneri many young men enjoy a woman that may be married to one of them, either one after the other, or at the same time. Thus one of them holds her, another enjoys her, a third uses her mouth, a fourth holds her middle part and in this way they go on enjoying her several parts alternately.

The same things can be done when several men are sitting in company with one courtesan, or when one courtesan is along with many men. In the same way, this can be done by the women of the king's harem when they accidentally get hold of a man .

The people in the southern countries have also a congress in the anus, that is called the 'lower congress.' (Ed. – Vatsyayana does not approve of sodomy.)

Thus end the various kinds of congress. There are also two verses on the subject as follows:

'An ingenious person should multiply the kinds of congress after the fashion of the different kinds of beasts and of birds. For these different kinds of congress, performed according to the usage of each country, and the liking of each individual, generate love, friendship, and respect in the hearts of women.'

Modes of Striking and Making Sounds of Passion

Sexual intercourse can be compared to a quarrel, on account of the contrarieties of love and its tendency of dispute. The place of striking with passion is the body, and on the body the special places are:

The shoulders

The back

The head

The *jaghana* or middle part of the body

The space between the breasts

The sides

Striking is of four kinds:

Striking with the back of the hand

Striking with the fist

Striking with the fingers a little contracted

Striking with the open palm of the hand

On account of its causing pain striking gives rise to the hissing sound, which is of various kinds, and to the eight kinds of crying:

The sound Hin

The sound Phut

The thundering sound

The sound Phat

The cooing sound

The sound Sut

The weeping sound

The sound Plat

Besides these, there are words having a meaning, such as 'mother' and those that are expressive of prohibition, sufficiency, desire of liberation, pain or praise, and to which may be added sounds like those of the dove, the cuckoo, the green pigeon, the parrot, the bee, the sparrow, the flamingo, the duck, and the quail, which are all occasionally made use of.

Blows with the fist should be given on the back of the woman, while she is sitting on the lap of the man, and she should give blows in return, abusing the man as if she were angry, and making the cooing and the weeping sounds. While the woman is engaged in congress, the space between the breasts should be struck with the back of the hand, slowly at first, and then proportionately to

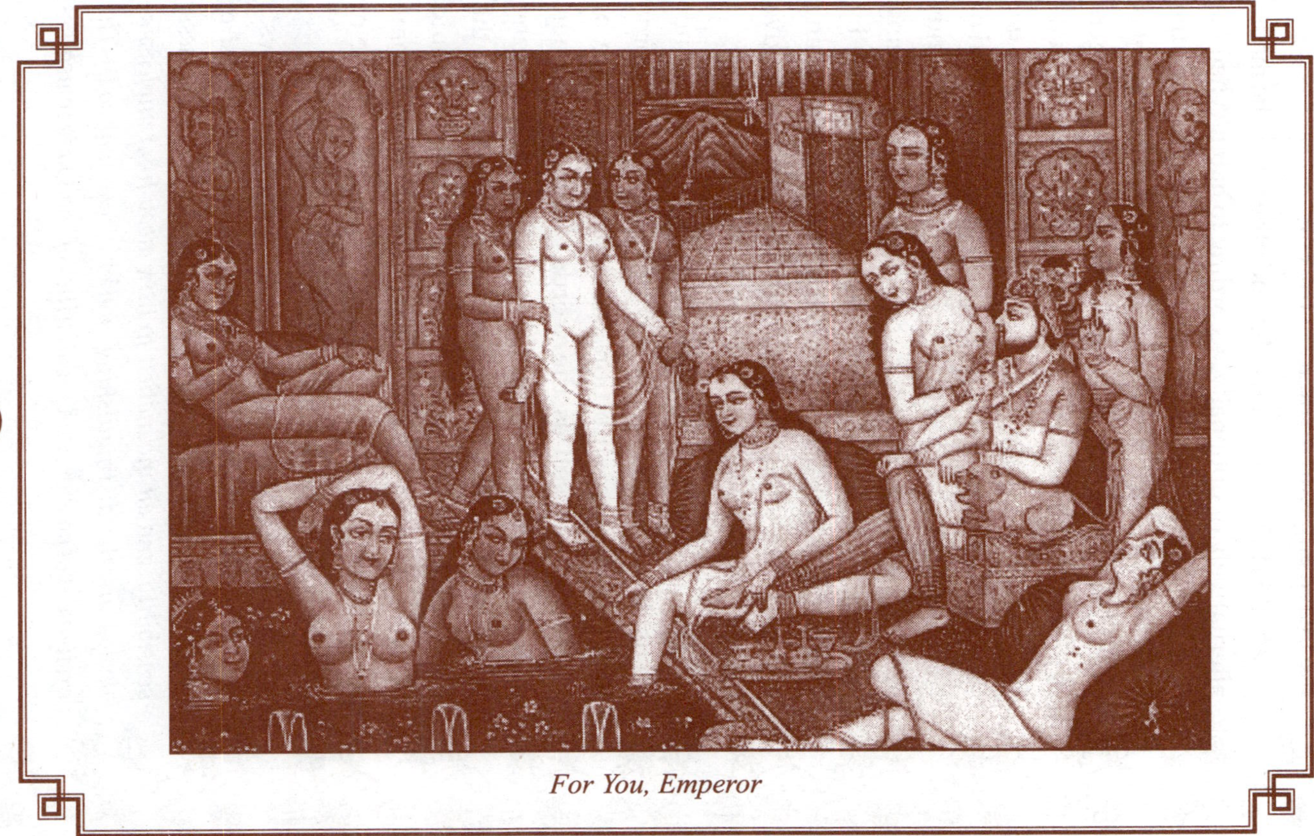

For You, Emperor

the increasing exitement, until the end.

At this time the sounds Hin and others may be made, alternatively or optionally, according to habit. When the man, making the sound Phat, strikes the woman on the head, with the finger of the hand a little contracted, it is called Prasritaka, which means striking with the fingers of the hand a little contracted. In this case the appropriate sounds are the cooing sounds, the sound Phat and the sound Phut in the interior of the mouth, and at the end of congress the sighing and weeping sounds. The sounds Phat is an imitation of the sound of a bamboo being split while the sound Phut is like the sound made by something falling into water. At all times when kissing and such like things are begun, the woman should give a reply with a hissing sound.

During the excitement when the woman is not accustomed to striking, she continually utters words expressive of prohibition, sufficiency or desire of liberation, as well as the words 'father', 'mother' intermingled with the sighing, weeping and thundering sounds. Towards the concluding of the congress, the breasts, the *jaghana*, and the sides of the woman should be pressed with the open palms of the hand, with some force, until the end of it, and then sounds like those of the quail or the goose should be made.

There are also two verses on the subject as follows:

'The characteristics of manhood are said to consist of roughness and impetuosity, while weakness, tenderness, sensibility, and an inclination to turn away from unpleasant things are the distinguishing marks of womanhood. The excitement of passion, and peculiarities of habit may sometimes

cause contrary results to appear, but these do not last long, and in the end the natural state is resumed.'

The wedge on the bosom, the scissors on the head, the piercing instrument on the cheeks, and the pinchers on the breasts and sides may also be taken into consideration with the other four modes of striking , and thus give eight ways altogether. But these four ways of striking with instruments are peculiar to the people of the southern countries, and the marks caused by them are seen on the breasts of their women. They are local peculiarities, but Vatsyayana is of opinion that the practice of them is painful, barbarous and base, and quite unworthy of imitation.

In the same way, anything that is a local peculiarity should not always be adopted elsewhere, and even in the place where the practice is prevalent, excess of it should always be avoided, Instances of the dangerous use of them may be given as follows:

The king of the Panchalas killed the courtesan Madhavasena by means of the wedge during congress. King Shatakarni of the Kuntalas deprived his great Queen Malayavati of her life by a pair of scissors, and Naradeva, whose hand was deformed, blinded a dancing girl by directing a piercing instrument in a wrong way.

There are also two verses on the subject as follows:

"About these things there cannot be either enumeration or any definite rule. Congress having once commenced, passion alone gives birth to all the acts of the parties.'

Such passionate actions and amorous gesticulations or movements which arise on the spur of the moment, and during sexual intercourse, cannot be defined, and are as irregular as dreams. A horse having once attained the fifth degree of motion goes on with blind speed, regardless of pits, ditches, and posts in his way; and in the same manner a loving pair become blind with passion in the heat of congress, and go on with great impetuosity paying not the least regard to excess of going. For this reason one who is well acquainted with the science of love, and knowing his own strength as also the tenderness, impetuosity, and strength of the young woman, should act accordingly. The various modes of enjoyment are not for all time or for all persons, but they should only be used at the proper time, and in proper countries and places.

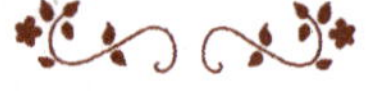

8
Women Acting as Man

When a woman sees that her lover is fatigued by constant congress, without having his desire satisfied, she should, with his permission, lay him down upon his back, and give him assistance by acting his part. She may also do this to satisfy that curiosity of her lover, or her own desire of novelty.

There are two ways of doing this, the first is when during congress she turns round and gets on the top of her lover, in such a manner as to continue the congress, without obstructing the pleasure of it; and the other is when she acts the man's part from the beginning. At such a time, with flowers in her hair hanging loose, and her smiles broken by hard breathings, she should press upon her lover's bosom with her own breasts, and lowering her head frequently should do in return the same actions which he used to do before, returning his blows and chaffing him, should say, 'I was laid down by you, and fatigued with hard congress, I shall now therefore lay you down in return'. She should then again manifest her own bashfulness, her fatigue, and her desire of stopping the congress. In this way, she should do the work of a man, which we shall presently relate.

Whatever is done by a man for giving pleasure to a woman is called the work of a man, and is as follows:

While the woman is lying on his bed, and is as it were

abstracted by his conversation, he should loosen the knot of her under- garments, and when she begins to dispute with him, he should overwhelm her with kisses. Then when his penis is erect, he should touch her with his hands in various places, and gently manipulate various parts of the body. If the woman is bashful, and if it is the first time that they have come together, the man should place his hands between her thighs, which she would probably keep close together, and if she is a very young girl, he should first get his hands upon her breasts, which she would probably cover with her own hands, and under her armpits and on her neck. If however she is a seasoned woman, he should do whatever is fitting for the occasion. After this he should take hold of her hair, and hold her chin in the fingers for the purpose of kissing her. On this, if she is a young girl, she will become bashful and close her eyes. Anyhow he should gather from the action of the woman what things would be pleasing to her during congress.

Suvarnanabha says that while a man is doing to the woman what he likes best during congress, he should always make a point of pressing those parts of her body on which she turns her eyes.

The signs of the enjoyment and satisfaction of the woman are as follows:

Let her body relax, she closes her eyes, she puts aside all bashfulness, and shows increased willingness to unite the two organs as closely together as possible.

On the other hand, the signs of her want of enjoyment and of failing to be satisfied are as follows:

She shakes her hands, she does not let the man get up, feels dejected, bites the man, kicks him, and continues to

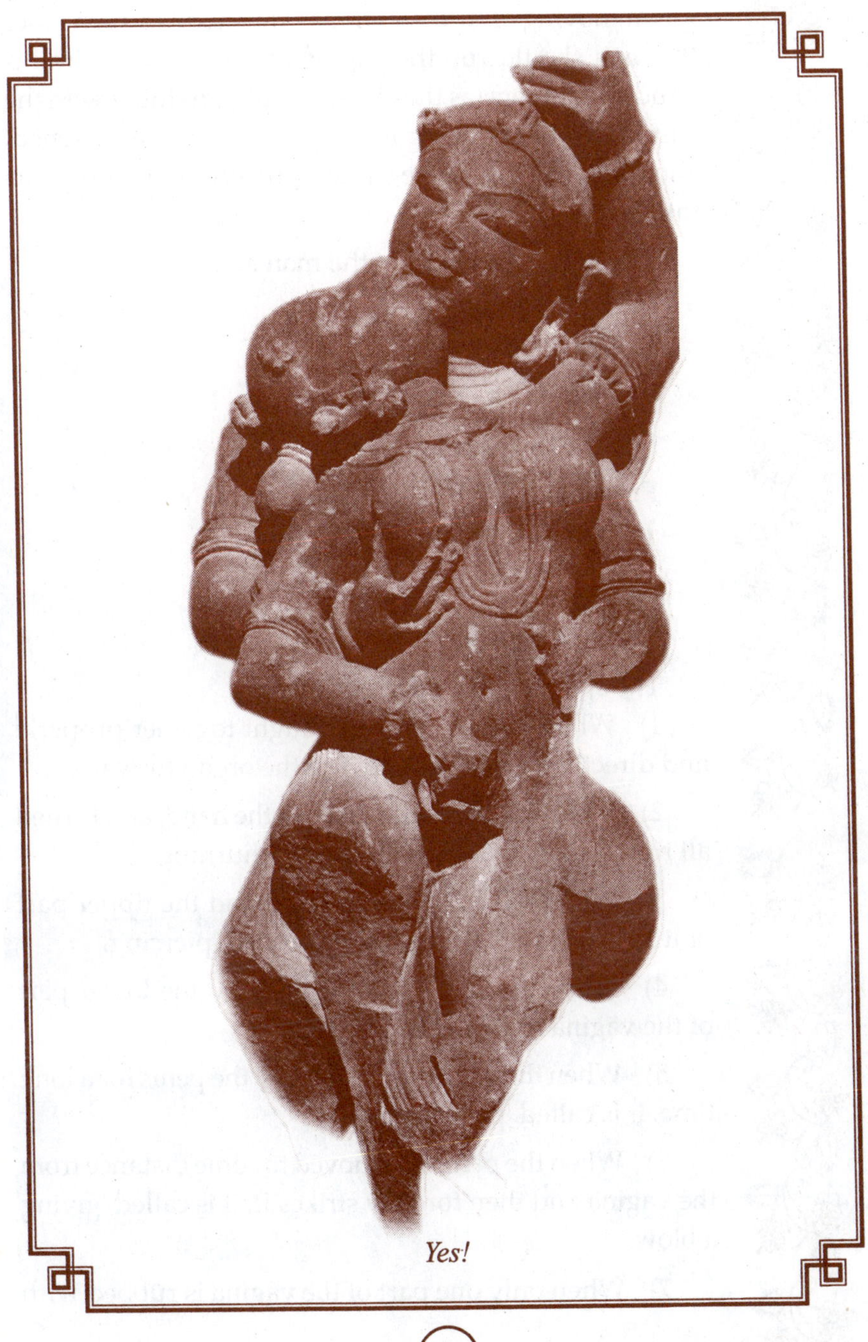

Yes!

go on moving after the man has finished. In such cases the man should rub the vagina of the woman with his hand and fingers (as the elephant rubs anything with the trunk) before engaging in congress, until it is softened, and after that is done he should proceed to put his penis into her.

The acts to be done by the man are:

Moving forward

Rubbing

The blow of a boar

Friction or churning

Pressing

The blow of a bull

Piercing

Giving a blow

The sporting of a sparrow

1) When the organs are brought together properly and directly it is called, 'moving the organ forward'.

2) When the penis is held with the hand, and turned all round in the vagina, it is called 'churning.'

3) When the vagina is lowered and the upper part of it is struck with the penis, it is called 'piercing.'

4) When the same thing is done on the lower part of the vagina it is called 'rubbing'.

5) When the vagina is pressed by the penis for a long time, it is called 'pressing'.

6) When the penis is removed to some distance from the vagina and then forcibly strikes it, it is called 'giving a blow.'

7) When only one part of the vagina is rubbed with

the penis it is called the 'blow of a boar'.

(8) When both sides of the vagina are rubbed in this way, it is called the 'blow of a bull'.

(9) When the penis is in the vagina, and is moved up and down frequently, and without being taken out, it is called the 'sporting of a sparrow'. This takes place at the end of congress.

When the woman acts the part of a man, she has the following things to do in addition to the nine given above:

The pair or tongs

The top

The swing

1) When the woman holds the penis in her vagina , draws it in, presses it, and keeps it thus in her for a long time, it is called the 'pair of tongs'.

2) When, while engaged, she turns round like a wheel, it is called the 'top.' This is learnt by practice only.

3) When, on such an occasion, the man lifts up the middle part of his body and the woman turns round her middle part, it is called the 'swing'.

When the woman is tired, she should place her forehead on that of her lover, and should thus take rest without disturbing the union of the organs, and when the woman has rested herself, the man should turn round and begin the congress again.

There are also some verses on the subject as follows:

'*Though a woman is reserved, and keeps her feelings*

concealed, yet when she gets on the top of a man, she then shows all her love and desire. A man should gather from the actions of the woman of what disposition she is, and in what way she likes to be enjoyed. A women during her monthly courses, a woman who has been lately confined, and a fat woman should not be made to act the part of a man.'

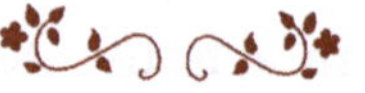

9
EUNUCHS AND THEIR ROLE

There are two kinds of eunuchs, those that are disguised as males, and those that are disguised as females. Eunuchs disguised as females imitate their dress, speech, gesture, tenderness, timidity, simplicity, softness and bashfulness. The acts that are done on the *jaghana* or middle parts of the woman, are done in the mouths of these eunuchs, and this is called Auparishtaka. These eunuchs derive their imaginative pleasure, and their livelihood from this kind of congress, and they lead the life of courtesans. So much concerning eunuchs disguised as females.

Eunuchs disguised as males keep their secret, and when they wish to anything, they lead the life of shampooers. Under the pretence of shampooing, an eunuch of this kind embraces and draws towards himself the things of the man whom he is shampooing, and after this he touches the joints of his thighs and his *jaghana* or central portion of his body. Then, if he finds the penis of the man erect, he presses it with his hands, and chaffs him for getting into that state; if after this, and after knowing his intention, the man does not tell the eunuch to proceed, then the latter does it of his own accord and brings the congress. If however he is ordered by the man to do it, then he disputes with him, and only consents at last with difficulty.

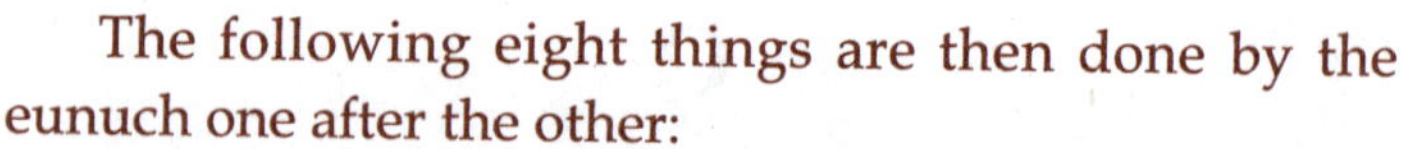

The following eight things are then done by the eunuch one after the other:

The nominal congress
Biting the sides
Pressing outside
Pressing inside
Kissing
Rubbing
Sucking a mango fruit
Swallowing up

At the end of each of these, the eunuch expresses his wish to stop, but when one of them is finished, the man desires him to do another, and after that is done, then the one that follows it and so on.

1) When, holding the man's penis with his hand, and placing it between his lips, the eunuch moves about his mouth, it is called the 'nominal congress'.

2) When, covering the end of the penis with his fingers collected together like the bud of a plant or flower, the eunuch presses the sides of it with his lips, using his teeth also, it is called 'biting the sides'.

3) When, being desired to proceed, the eunuch presses the end of the penis with his lips closed together, and kisses it as if he were drawing it out, it is called 'the outside pressing'.

4) When, being asked to go on he puts the penis further into his mouth, and presses it with his lips and then takes it out it is called the 'inside pressing'.

5) When, holding the penis in his hand, the eunuch kisses it as if he were kissing the lower lip, it is called 'kissing'.

6) When, after kissing it, he touches it with his tongue everywhere and passes the tongue over the end of it, it is called 'rubbing'.

7) When, in the same way, he puts the half of it into his mouth and forcibly kisses and sucks it, this is called 'sucking a mango fruit.'

8) And lastly, when, with the consent of the man, the eunuch puts the whole penis into his mouth, and presses it to the very end, as if he were going to swallow it up, it is called 'swallowing it up'.

Striking, scratching, and other things may also be done during this kind of congress.

The Auparishtaka is practiced also by unchaste and wanton women, female attendants and serving maids, i.e., those who are not married to anybody, but who live by shampooing.

The Acharyas are of opinion that this Auparishtaka is the work of a dog and not of a man, because it is a low practice, and opposed to the orders of the scriptures and because the man himself suffers by bringing his penis into contact with the mouths of eunuchs and women. But Vatsyayana says that the orders of scriptures do not affect those who resort to courtesans, and the law prohibits the practice of the Auparishtaka with married women only. As regards the injury to the male, that can be easily remedied.

Practices in Various Lands

The people of Eastern India do not resort to women who practise the Auparishtaka.

The people of Ahichhatra resort of such women, but do nothing with them so far as the mouth is concerned.

The people of Saket (Ayodhya) do with these women every kind of mouth congress, while the people of Nagara do not practise this, but do every other thing.

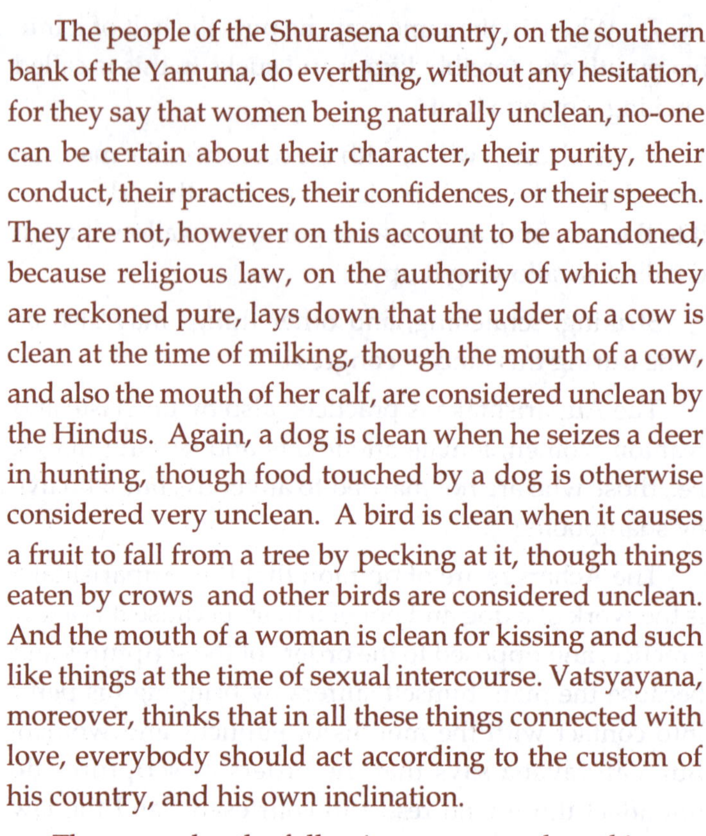

The people of the Shurasena country, on the southern bank of the Yamuna, do everthing, without any hesitation, for they say that women being naturally unclean, no-one can be certain about their character, their purity, their conduct, their practices, their confidences, or their speech. They are not, however on this account to be abandoned, because religious law, on the authority of which they are reckoned pure, lays down that the udder of a cow is clean at the time of milking, though the mouth of a cow, and also the mouth of her calf, are considered unclean by the Hindus. Again, a dog is clean when he seizes a deer in hunting, though food touched by a dog is otherwise considered very unclean. A bird is clean when it causes a fruit to fall from a tree by pecking at it, though things eaten by crows and other birds are considered unclean. And the mouth of a woman is clean for kissing and such like things at the time of sexual intercourse. Vatsyayana, moreover, thinks that in all these things connected with love, everybody should act according to the custom of his country, and his own inclination.

There are also the following verses on the subject:

'The male servants of some men carry on the mouth-congress with their masters. It is also practised by some citizens, who know each other well, among themselves, Some women of the harem, when they are amorous, do the acts of the mouth on the vaginas of one another, and some men do the same things with women. The way of doing this (kissing the vagina) should be known from kissing the mouth. When a man and woman lie down in an inverted order, with the head of the one towards the feet of the other, and carry on this congress, it is called the congress of a crow.'

For the sake of such things, courtesans abandon

men possessed of good qualities, liberal and clever, and become attached to low persons, such as slaves and elephant-drivers. The Auparishtaka, or mouth-congress, should never be done by a learned Brahman, by a minister that carried on the business of a state, or by a man of good reputation, because though the practice is allowed by the shastras, there is no reason why it should be carried on, and need only be practised in particular cases.

As for instance the taste, and the strength, and the digestive qualities of the flesh of dogs are mentioned in works on medicine, but it does not therefore follow that it should be eaten by the wise. In the same way, there are some men, some places and some times, with respect of which these practices can be made use of. A man should therefore pay regard to the place, to the time, and to the practice which is to be carried out, as also to whether it is agreeable to his nature and to himself, and then he may or may not practise these things according to circumstances. But after all, these things being done secretly, and the mind of the man being fickle, how can it be known what any person will do at any particular time and for any particular purpose.

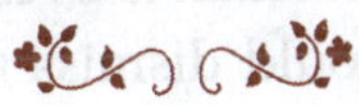

10
The Kinds of Sexual Union & Love-Quarrels

In the pleasure-room, decorated with flowers, and fragrant with perfumes, attended by his friends and servants, the citizen should receive the woman, who will come bathed and dressed, and will invite her to take refreshment and to drink freely. He should then seat her on his left side, and holding her hair, and touching also the end and knot of her garment, he should gently embrace her with his right arm. They should then carry on an amusing conversation on various subjects, and may also talk suggestively of things which would be considered as coarse, or not to be mentioned generally in society. They may then sing, either with or without gesticulations, and ply on musical instruments, talk about the arts, and persuade each other to drink.

At last when the woman is overcome with love and desire, the citizen should dismiss the people that may be with him, giving them flowers, ointments, and betel leaves, and then when the two are left alone, they should proceed as has been already described in the previous chapters.

Such is the beginning of sexual union. At the end of the congress, the lovers, with modesty, and not looking at each other, should go separately to the washing-room. After this, sitting in their own places, they should eat some betel leaves, and the citizen should apply with his own hand to the body of the woman some pure sandalwood ointment, or ointment of some other kind. He should then embrace her with his left arm, and with agreeable words should cause her to drink from a cup held in his own hand, or he may give her water to drink. They can then eat sweetmeats or anyting else, according to their liking, and may drink fresh juice, soup, gruel, extracts of meat, *sherbet* , the juice of mango fruits, the extract of the juice of the citron tree mixed with sugar, or anything that may be liked in different countires, and known to be sweet, soft, and pure. The lovers may also sit on the terrace of the palace or house, and enjoy the moonlight, and carry on an agreeable conversation. At this time too, while the woman lies in his lap, with her face towards the moon, the citizen should show her the different planets, the morning star, the polar star, and the seven Rishis, or Great Bear.

This is the end of sexual union.

The congress is of the following kinds:
Loving congress

Congress like that of eunuchs

Congress of subsequent love

Deceitful congress

Congress of artificial love

Congress of spontaneous love

Congress of transferred love

1) When a man and a woman, who have been in love with each other for some time, come together with great difficulty, or when one of the two returns from a journey, or is reconciled after having been separated on account of a quarrel, then congress is called the 'loving

Congress'. It is carried on according to the liking of the lovers, and as long as they choose.

2) When two persons come together, while their love for each other is still in its infancy, their congress is called the 'congress of subsequent love'.

3) When a man carries on the congress by exciting himself by means of the sixty-four ways, such as kissing, etc., etc., or when a man and a woman come together, though in reality they are both attached to different persons, their congress is then called the 'congress of artificial love'. At this time all the ways and means mentioned in the Kama Shastra should be used.

4) When a man, from the beginning to the end of the congress, though having connection with the woman, thinks all the time that he is enjoying another one whom he loves, it is called the 'congress of transferred love.'

5) The congress between a man and a female water -carrier, or a female servant of a caste lower than his own, lasting only until the desire is satisfied, is called the 'congress like that of eunuchs'. Here external touches, kisses and manipulations are not to be employed.

6) The congress between a courtesan and a rustic, and that between citizens and the women of villages, and bordering countries, is called 'deceitful congress.'

7) The congress that takes place between two persons who are attached to one another, and which is done according to their own liking, is called 'spontaneous congress'.

Thus ends the kinds of congress.

Love Quarrels

We shall now speak of love quarrels.

A woman who is very much in love with a man cannot bear to hear the name of her rival mentioned, or to have any conversation regarding her, or to be addressed by her name through a mistake. If such a thing takes place, a great quarrel arises, and the woman cries, becomes angry, tosses her hair about, strikes her lover, falls from her bed or seat, and casting aside her garlands and ornaments, throws herself down on the ground.

At this time, the lover should attempt to reconcile her with conciliatory words, and should take her up carefully and place her on her bed. But she, not replying to his questions, and with increased anger, should bend down his head by pulling his hair, and having kicked him once, twice or thrice on his arms, head, bosom or back, should then proceed to the door of the room. Dattaka says that she should then sit angrily near the door and shed tears, but should not go out, because she would be found at fault with for going away. After a time, when she thinks that the conciliatory words and actions of her lover have reached their utmost, she should then embrace him, talking to him with harsh and reproachful words, but at the same time showing a loving desire for congress.

When a woman is in her own house, and has quarrelled with her lover, she should go to him and show how angry she is, and leave him. Afterwards the citizen having sent the Vita, the Vidushaka or the Pithamarda to pacify her, she should accompany them back to the house, and spend the night with her lover.

Thus end the love quarrels.

A man, employing the sixty-four means mentioned by Babhravya, obtains his object, and enjoys the woman of the first quality. Though he may speak well on other

subjects, if he does not know the sixty-four divisions, no great respect is paid to him in the assembly of the learned. A man, devoid of other knowledge, but well acquainted with the sixty-four divisions becomes a leader in any society of men and women. What man will not respect the sixty-four arts, considering they are respected by the learned, by the cunning, and by the courtesans. As the sixty-four arts are respected, are charming, and add to the talent of women, they are called by the Acharyas dear to women. A man skilled in the sixty-four arts is looked upon with love by his own wife, by the wives of others, and by courtesans.

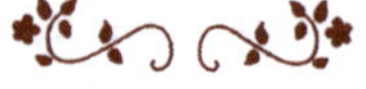

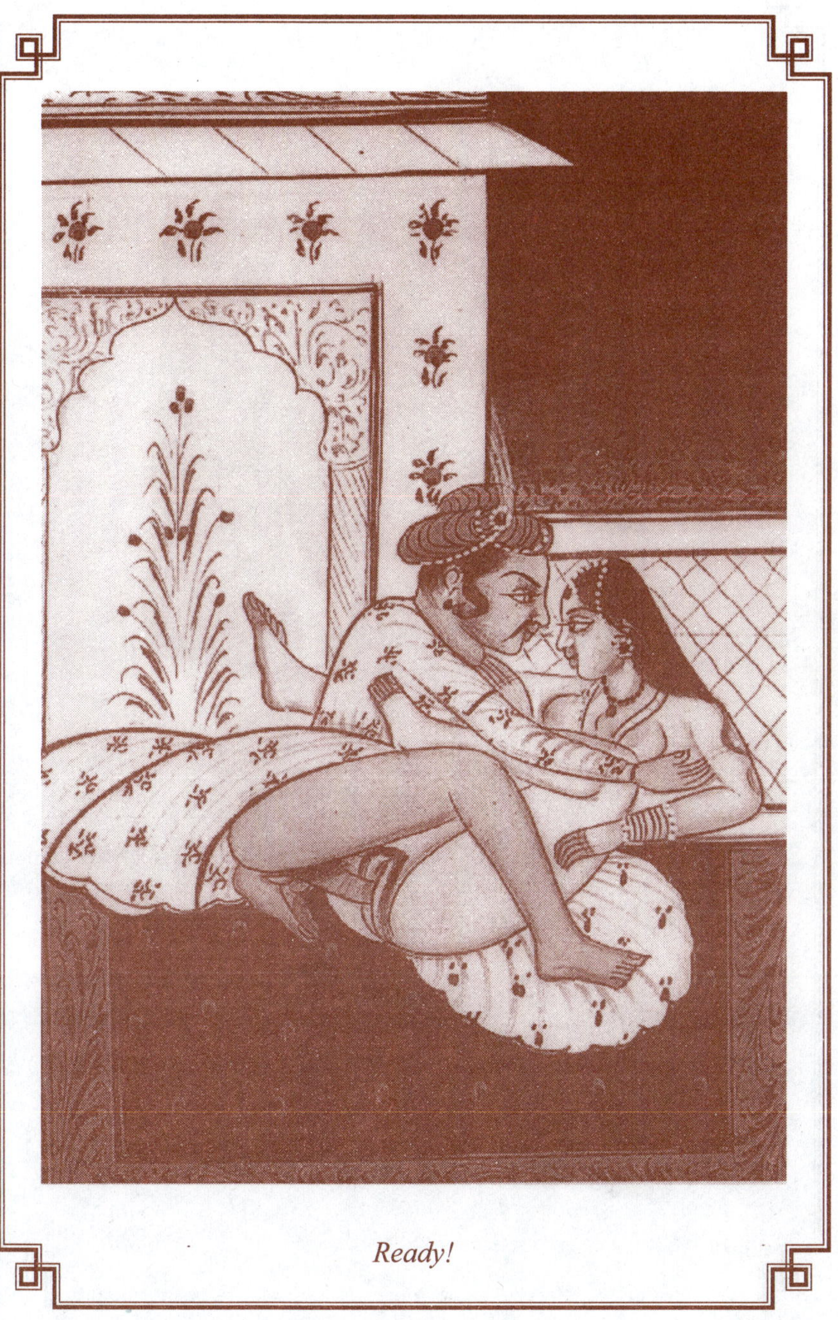

Ready!

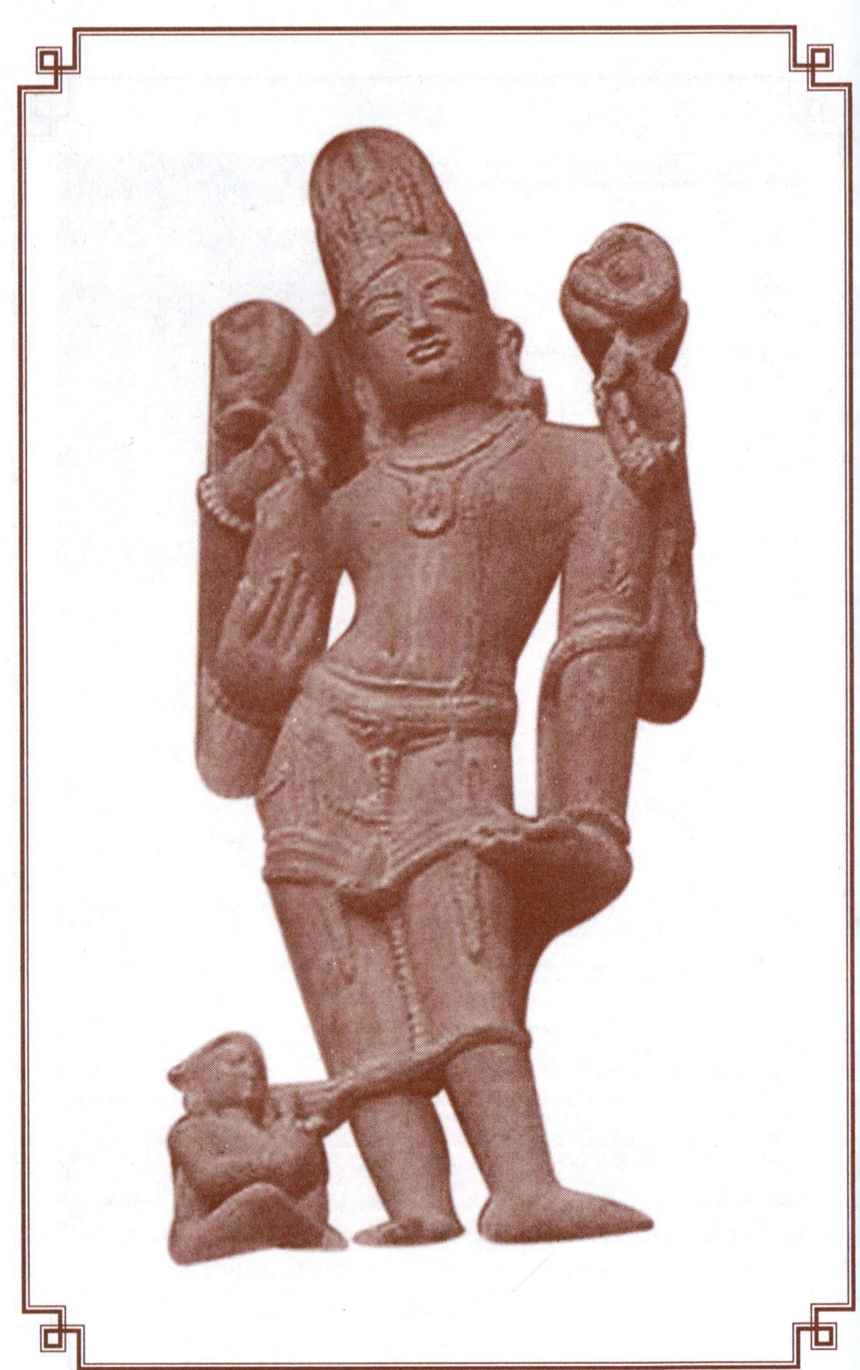

3

INDIAN LIFE IN THE TIMES OF VATSYAYANA

H.C. CHAKLADAR

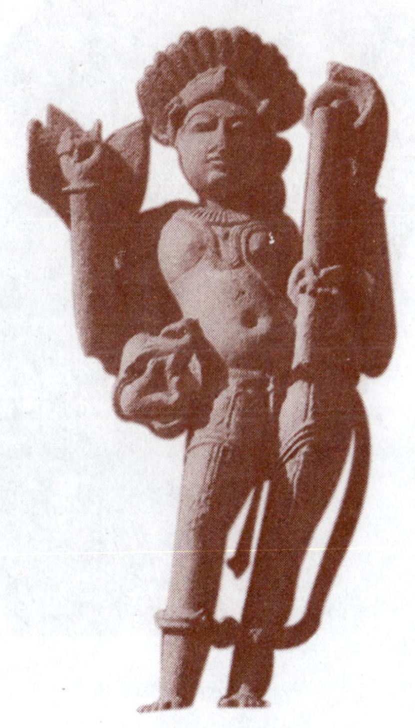

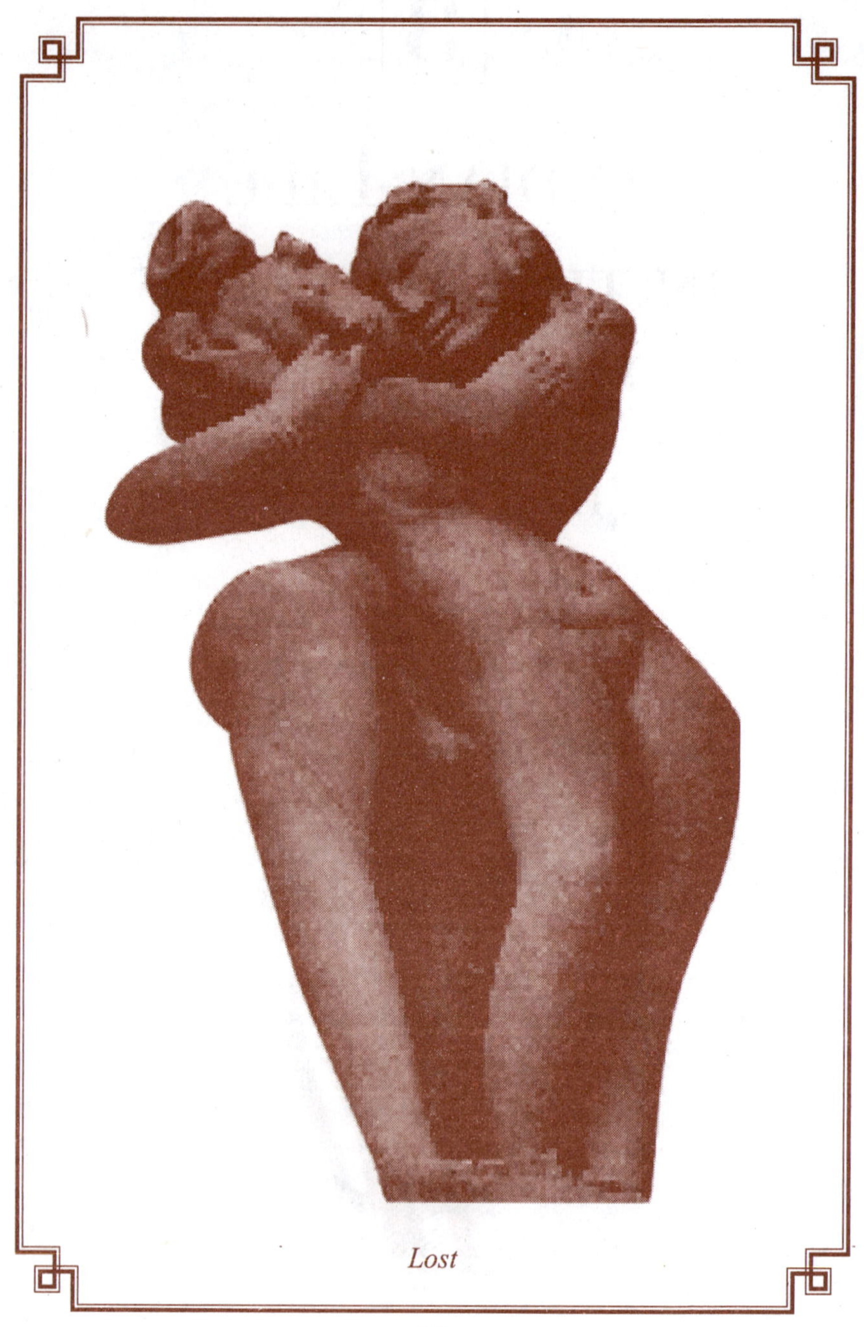

Lost

1

THE BACKGROUND OF KAMASUTRA

Vatsyayana stands pre-eminent in early Indian literature as an author who brought the analytical power of a keen logician to bear on the science of erotics which, in our modern days, has only lately begun to be studied with the care that it deserves. The science had attracted the serious attention of the Indian savants very early, as far back, perhaps, as the time when the 'Satapatha Brahmana' was being compiled, and in the centuries that elapsed before Vatsyayana made his appearance, the various sections of the science were being studied separately and individually. But it was Vatsyayana who synthesized the whole science and revived the popular interest in this branch of knowledge. Apart from its interest in a work on the science of love, Vatsyayana's Kamasutra is of immense importance to us as throwing a flood of light on the manners and customs of his contemporary Indian society.

In speaking of the origin of the Kamasutra, Vatsyaynana says at the beginning of his work that at first Prajapati, the 'Lord of beings' for the welfare and preservation of the progeny composed a huge encyclopaedia in hundred thousand chapters dealing with the three objects of human life, viz., dharma, artha and kama,; the first two of these subjects were next taken up by Manu and Brihaspati respectively, and Nandi, the attendant of Mahadeva, took up the third which he dealt with in a thousand chapters. This last work was condensed into five hundred chapters by Shvetaketu, the son of Uddalaka. The work of Shvetaketu was further abridged into a hundred and fifty chapters and divided into seven sections by Babhravya, a native of the Panchala country. Next, Dattaka, at the request of the courtesans of Pataliputra, wrote a separate treatise dealing with the Vahisika section of Babhravya. His example was followed by six other writers – Charayana, Suvarnanabha, Ghotakamukha, Gonardiya, Gonikaputra and Kuchumara, each of whom took up a section of Babhravya and wrote a monograph on it.

As the science treated in this fragmentary fashion by numerous writers was about to be mangled and spoiled and as the work of Babhravya, being huge in bulk, was difficult to be mastered, Vatsyayana proposed to give an epitome of the whole subject in a single work of moderate dimensions. Towards the end of the Kamasutra, again, Vatsyayana says that having from his teachers, as one would do in the case of a sacred text of Agama and having pondered over them in his mind, he composed the Kamasutra in the approved method. He thus admits that the great work of Babhravya formed the groundwork of his own book as is also quite evident form the frequent reference that he makes to it in every part of his Kamasutra: one out of his seven sections, the Samproyogika, covering about a fourth part of the whole work, is entirely taken from Babhravya, as he says at the end of that section.

It may be noted that Vatsyayana speaks of having treated Babhravya's book like an Agama, a work of holy scripture, indicating that it was considerably ancient. A Babhravya who is called Panchala by Uvata, the commentator, is mentioned in the Rig-pratishakhya as the author of the Kramapatha of the Rigveda and

Professor Weber holds that this Babhravya Panchala, and the Panchala people through him, took a leading part in fixing and arranging the text of the Rigveda.

The Panchala country where Babhravya flourished appears to have been the part of India where the science of erotics was specially cultivated. The Panchala people were evidently credited in ancient times with special knowledge in matters relating to the sexes, and one of them is said to have changed even the natural sex, as we see in the case of hikhandin, the son of the Panchala king, Drupada. Polyandry as we see it in the case of Draupadi Panchali, may be regarded as an ancient institution of the Panchala country, and the Pandava brothers, belonging as they did, to the allied tribe of the Kurus, as we see from the common Vedic phrase Kuru-Panchala, were certainly familiar with it and could have no difficulty in acceding to it.

In this connection, a statement of Vatsyayana is very significant. He says that according to the followers of Babhravya, a woman's chastity may not be respected when she is found to have intimacy with five lovers (in addition to her husband, explains the commentary), showing that five was considered as the limit beyond which it was not proper for a woman to go; if she did so, she should be approached with impunity by anyone. The commentary explains that in the case of Draupadi this limit was not passed, as Yudhishthira and others were all her husbands. The indulgence shown by the Panchala people to five lovers, appears to be significant.

The author of the Kamasutra is mentioned by name in the 'Vasavadatta' of Subandhu who is supposed to have flourished about the same time as Chandragupta

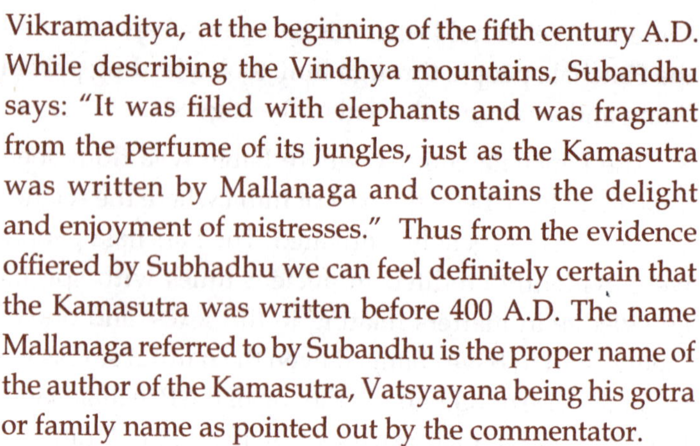

Vikramaditya, at the beginning of the fifth century A.D. While describing the Vindhya mountains, Subandhu says: "It was filled with elephants and was fragrant from the perfume of its jungles, just as the Kamasutra was written by Mallanaga and contains the delight and enjoyment of mistresses." Thus from the evidence offiered by Subhadhu we can feel definitely certain that the Kamasutra was written before 400 A.D. The name Mallanaga referred to by Subandhu is the proper name of the author of the Kamasutra, Vatsyayana being his gotra or family name as pointed out by the commentator.

We thus see that the earlier limit to the composition of the Kamasutra may be assigned on the basis of Vatsyayana's quotations, from the Grhya and Dharma Sutras the Arthashastra' of Kautilya nd the 'Mahabhashya' of Patanjali and that the lower limit may be fixed at 400 A.D. based on the dates of Kalidasa and Subandhu and, further, that there are strong reasons to believe that it was known in the third century A.D.

The conclusion is inevitable that the Kamasutra was composed about the middle of the third century A.D.

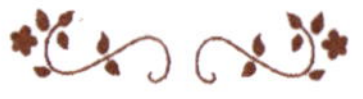

2
LIFE IN THE CITIES

Vatsyayana in his work holds up the ideal of city-life. He wrote the Kamasutra as a practical handbook for the guidance of city bred men of fashion – the Nagarakas. A whole section of his book is called Nagaraka-vrittam, wherein he describes the life of a city-man, not of a mere dweller in a city—such a person would only be a Nagara—but of a Nagaraka, who, according to Panini, is a city bred man skilled in the arts and knaveries that specially develop in a big city, one possessing the virtues and vices of a "a cockney" he might be a clever artist or a knave, as the 'Kahika-vritti' so naively explains.

Vatsyayana's book is calculated to benefit such men and women, among them princesses and daughters of high officials (Mahamatras), who armed with an expert knowledge of the practical directions given by him, would be able to subdue the heart of a husband whose love is shared by a crowded harem of as many as a "thousand" wives. Vatsyayana recommends the city as the proper place of abode for a person who after finishing his education, thinks of entering the world, the Grihasthashrama, with the wealth that he may have acquired, either by inheritance or by the pursuit of the profession particularly appertaining to his own caste and his position in society; such a man should adopt the life of a Nagaraka and fix his habitation in a city—whether small or big, a *nagara*, or a *pattana*, or a *kharvata*, or at least

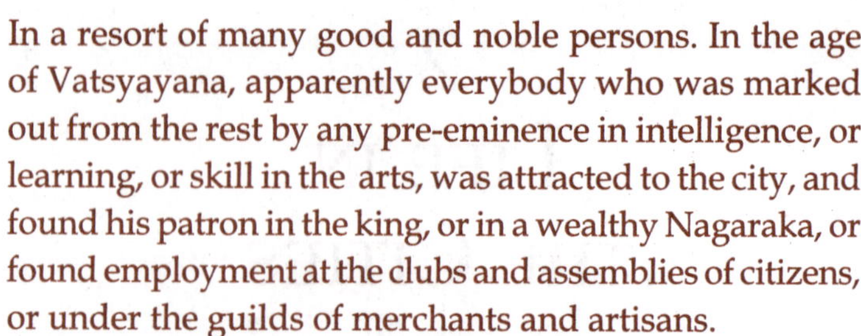

In a resort of many good and noble persons. In the age of Vatsyayana, apparently everybody who was marked out from the rest by any pre-eminence in intelligence, or learning, or skill in the arts, was attracted to the city, and found his patron in the king, or in a wealthy Nagaraka, or found employment at the clubs and assemblies of citizens, or under the guilds of merchants and artisans.

The City-bred Man of Fashion

If a person could not afford to live in a city and was forced to shut himself up in a village by the exigencies of earning his livelihood, even then he should, according to Vatsyayana, look upon civic life as the ideal and by giving to his fellow villagers glowing descriptions of the pleasant life led by the Nagaraka, he should inspire those among his own class who show any special cleverness or curiosity, with a desire to imitate the conduct of the city-people and he should give them a taste of the amenities of city-life by starting clubs and social gatherings as in the city, by himself gratifying his friends with his company, by favouring them with his assistance and by introducing the spirit of mutual help and co-operation. A village-wife is spoken of as a simpleton and village-women generally are spoken of as very light and fickle; such rustic women are regarded with scant courtesy by Vatsyayana.

The life of a round of pleasures in the city was naturally very expensive and many ran through their fortunes. Such a Nagaraka who had eaten up his fortune might, however, if clever, earn a living by placing himself at the service of the clubs and pleasure-houses where he would be respected on account of his skill in the arts, and then he would be called a *vita*. Even if a man had no fortune of his own he might enjoy the pleasures of life as a *pithamarda*; he might acquire skill in the arts and go about

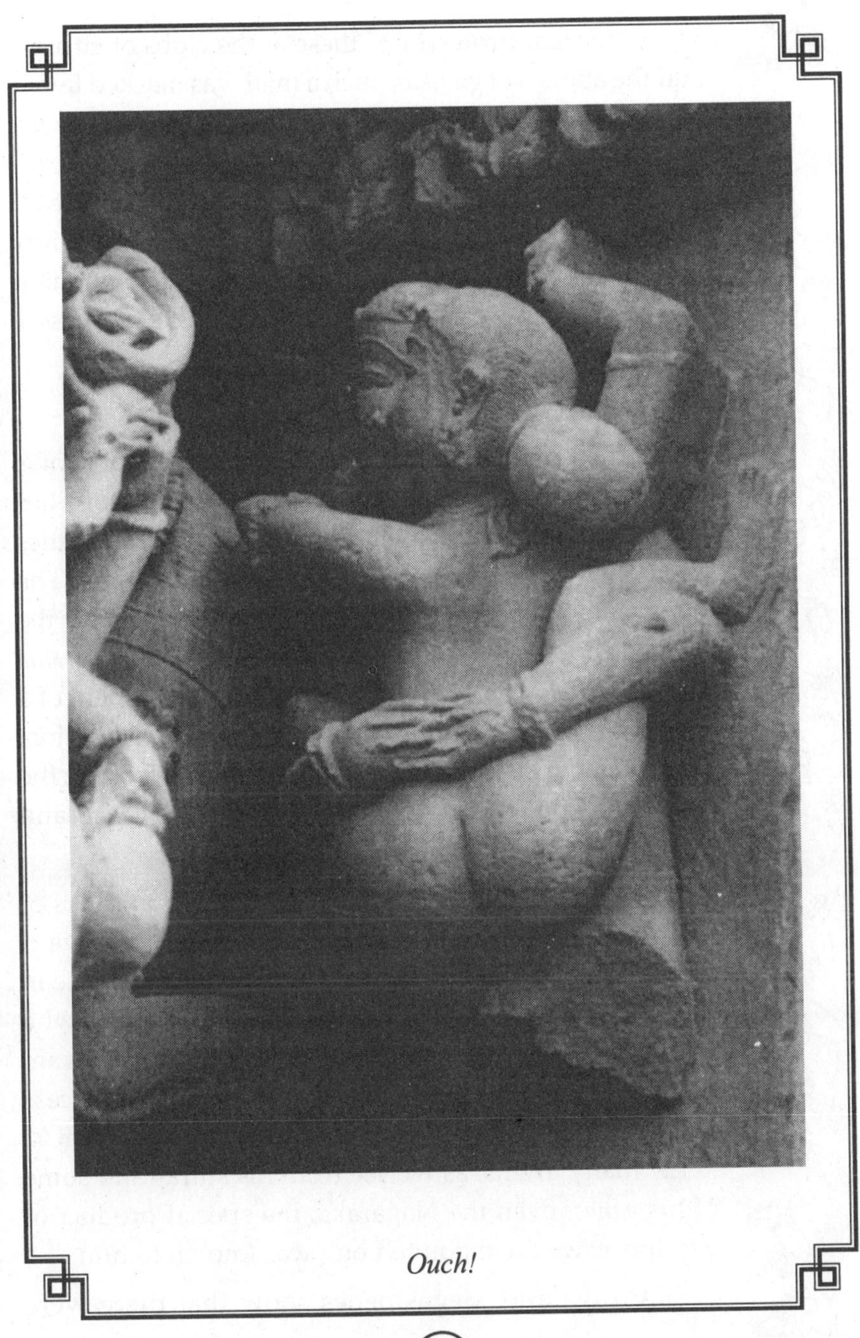

Ouch!

as an itinerant professor of these at the clubs of citizens and the abodes of *ganikas;* such a man was marked by his peculiar seat (*mallika*) which he hung on his back, by his dyed clothes and by some kind of soap (*phenaka*) which he always carried about in order to keep himself clean. Or he might, if he was skilled in only a few of the arts attach himself to a wealthy Nagaraka as his companion and confidential friend and then he was called a *vidusaka* or a *vaihasika,* a professional jester.

Growth of Cities

This strong desire for the gay life of the city shows that there must have been a pretty large number of cities at the time when Vatsyayana's work was written. Cities had grown up in India from very ancient times. The village and its headman are no doubt often met with in the Rigveda but the *grama* sometimes grew into a *mahagrama* and people naturally crowded round the settlement of a powerful chieftain, round his *pura* or fortified habitation. In later Vedic literature, cities were very well known; the 'Manava Grihyasutra' mentions the *grama,* the *nagara* and the *nigama.*

The cities were very well known to the compilers of the Dharmasutras, Baudhayana going so far as to warn people desirous of spiritual growth against residence in cities: he declares that it is hardly possible for a man who resides in a town – "whose body, whose face and eyes are defiled by the impure dust of a city":-- to obtain success in his spiritual quest. Panini in the seventh century B.C. knew many towns, as we see from his sutras and some of his *ganas,* even the Nagaraka, the special product of city-life as we have pointed out, was known to him.

Kautilya and Megasthenes show that there were

some very big cities with elaborate arrangements for civic government and that municipal organization of the city had developed wonderfully. In the Jatakas and the Buddhist Pali texts we find the description of large and prosperous cities which were seats of government and where trade flourished, where the *gahapati* was a prominent citizen and the *sresthi* took a leading part. The 'Milinda Panho' gives a splendid description of the town of Sakala, and nearer Vatsyayana's time, we find beautiful descriptions of splendid and prosperous towns given in the 'Buddhacharita' and 'Lalitavistara'. In Vatsyayana's time all over India there must have been a large number of cities, great and small, for India was then broken up into innumerable principalities and each prince had his own fortified capital. Besides, cities had grown up at places of pilgrimage – Brahmanic, Buddhist and Jain – or had sprung up as centres of the growing trade of the country. It was for the dwellers of these cities, where wealth accumulated and where the virtues and vices that wealth brings in its train specially developed, that Vatsyayana wrote his great work.

Economic Prosperity

At the time that Vatsyayana wrote India was carrying on an abundant trade, by land and by sea, with China on the one hand and the Roman orient on the other. According to a Chinese book 'Funantu-suhtchuan' written in the third century, Kuntien or Kaundinya founded an Indian colony in Indo-China about B.C. 53, and it soon grew up into a great centre of foreign trade in that quarter. By way of this Brahmanic colony planted in Indo-China, the Indians carried on an ever-increasing maritime trade with China in the approved Chinese method of sending so called embassies and making an exchange of presents.

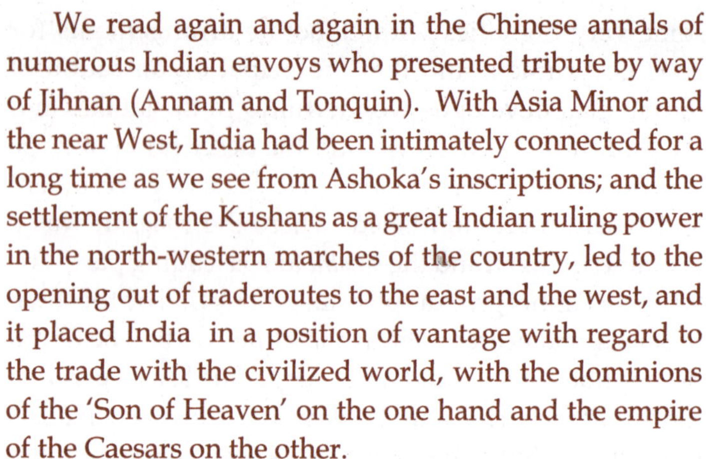

We read again and again in the Chinese annals of numerous Indian envoys who presented tribute by way of Jihnan (Annam and Tonquin). With Asia Minor and the near West, India had been intimately connected for a long time as we see from Ashoka's inscriptions; and the settlement of the Kushans as a great Indian ruling power in the north-western marches of the country, led to the opening out of traderoutes to the east and the west, and it placed India in a position of vantage with regard to the trade with the civilized world, with the dominions of the 'Son of Heaven' on the one hand and the empire of the Caesars on the other.

When in the second century A.D. not very long before Vatsyayana, a great Kushan emperor adopted the magnificent title of 'Maharaja-Rajatiraja-Devaputra-Kaisara Kanishka—'The great king, the king of kings, the son of heaven, the Caesar Kanishka,' we see that in him there was a fusion of the three great civilizations of the time—the Indian, the Chinese and the Roman. The currency of the Kushans shows an equally international character and seems to be designed to facilitate the trade of these dominions with the rest of the world; the coins show a strange and wonderful combination of Greek, Zoroastrian and Indian designs and icons; some of them have Jupiter on one side and Buddha on the other; they have legends in Greek, Iranian or Indian vernaculars and in varied scripts, Greek, Brahmi or Kharosthi. There cannot be any doubt that these coins were intended for currency inside as well as outside and they afforded facility of exchange to the Indian merchants trading with the near West.

Vatsyayana also knew coins of copper, silver and gold. He speaks of a *karsapana* of small value of the *niska* or coin of gold; besides, he refers to the art of examining *rupyas* or coins as one of the sixty-four *kalas*. Moreover, he uses the word *hiranya* to mean money in general including, perhaps, gold and silver coins.

Pliny in the first cenutry and Ptolemy in the second, testify to the great trade that India had with the Roman empire. In the third century when Vatsyayana lived, this trade must have gone on increasing and we shall not be far mistaken to conjecture that the Brahmanic colonies that Fa Hien visited in Java, went out about this period. The prosperity that this extensive commerce with the civilised world conferred on India, is fully reflected in the life of the Nagaraka, everything about whom, his house and furniture , address and ornaments, sports and pastimes, charity and liberality, bespeak an unstinted expenditure of wealth.

The literature of the period to which Vatsyayana belongs, amply corroborates the description that he gives of society. But we shall have room only to quote an occasional passage here and there from the works of Bhasa and from the 'Lalitavistara' both of which are supposed to belong to the third century and, therefore, to have been written about the same time as the Kamasutra; we may also draw some illustrations from the works of Ashvaghosa who flourished about a century earlier and belongs virtually to the same epoch.

The House of a City-bred Man

The house that the Nagaraka builds for his residence shows his taste and love of beauty and the simple but choice furniture and decoration that adorn his rooms show his love of art and his manysided culture. As we have seen before, the Nagaraka builds his house in a city.

It has to be in close proximity to a supply of water and divided into two parts, the inner belonging to the ladies and the outer where, as we shall see, the master of the house attends to business and receives visitors.

There is a number of rooms each set apart for its special purpose, and attached to the house there must be a garden with wide grounds, if possible, where flowering plants and fruit-trees can grow as well as kitchen vegetables. In the middle of the ground should be excavated either a well, or if there is room enough, a tank or a lake. This garden is attached to the inner court and is looked after by the mistress of the house. It is the duty of a good housewife, says Vatsyayana, to procure the seeds of the common Indian kitchen vegetables and medicinal herbs and plant them each in its season. In neat and clean spots in the garden where the ground has been well dressed, the lady of the house plants beds of green vegetables, clumps of the tall sugarcane, patches of stunted shrubs of the mustard and similar herbs, and thickets of the dark *tamala*.

The flower-garden equally receives her tender care; she has to see that it is laid out with beds of plants that yield an abundance of flowers — those that regale the nose with their sweet perfume, like the *mallika*, the *jati* or the *navamallika*, as well as those that delight the eye like the *japa* with its crimson glory or the *kurantaka* (amaranth) with its unfading yellow splendour, and besides, there should be in this garden, rows of shrubs yielding fragrant leaves or roots, like *bilaka* and *ustra*. In the gardens there are arbors and sometimes vine-groves where she gets built *sthandilas* or raised platforms with pleasant and comfortable seats for rest or recreation. Flowers should be spread on these seats in these sweet syluan retreats

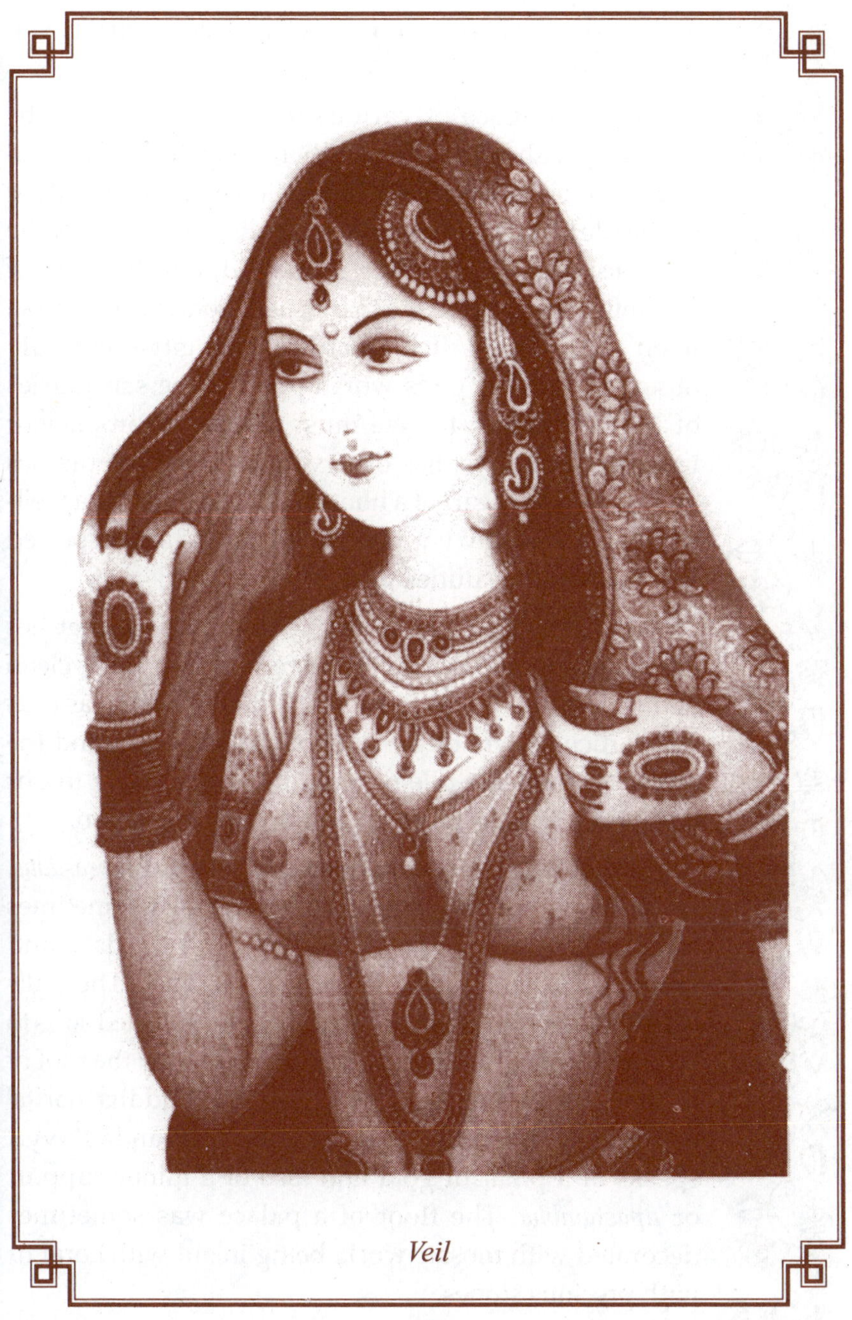

Veil

and a swing be hung at a spot well guarded from the sun by its leafy arbor.

An abundance of various flowers should also be arranged with art, here and there over the residential house which must be kept scrupulously clean, the floor should be beautifully smooth and polished so as to soothe the eyes; besides attending to these duties, the lady of the house should also see that at her abode the morning, noon and evening rites—sacrifices and gifts—are duly observed and the gods worshipped at the sanctuaries of the household; for we must realize, as an ancient teacher, Gonardiya, has observed, that nothing pleases and charms the heart of a householder so much as a well-kept, neat and tidy home where the gods are respected and the religious duties well observed.

The mistress of the house should also see that her kitchen is situated in a quiet and retired spot and is clean and attractive. The proper keeping of the house was thus the particular care of the wife of the Nagaraka and the erection of a noble pile of building is, according to our author, among the most earnest desires of women.

Large and magnificent houses; *harmyas* and *prasadas*, were known to Vatsyayana, the Nagaraka sometimes might enjoy moonlight on the terrace of a palace and examine the stars and planets with his beloved. The walls of the houses were sometimes beautifully polished so as to reflect the image of a girl, and not infrequently the roof of the house stood on pillars, *stambhas*. The 'Buddhacharita' mentions an iron pillar and the 'Saundarananda Kavya' speaks of a pillar of gold and also of a minor support or *upastambha*. The floor of a palace was sometimes decorated with mosaic work, being inlaid with coral or with precious stones.

In the palace-gardens there were *samudra-grihas* or cool summer houses surrounded by water, washed as it were, by the sea, and also rooms in the walls of which there were secret passages for water to circulate and take away the heat. Bhasa's 'Svapna-vasavadattam'. (Act-V) has such a samudragriha, and in later dramas also it is not rare; the '*Visnusmriti*' prescribes punishment for a *samudragriha-bhedaka*. Secret pleasure-houses standing amidst the waters of garden-tanks are referred to by Kalidasa. 'Besides the garden' Vatsyayana has not given much detailed description of the *antahpura* or the inner sanctum of the ladies. Bhasa designates it as the inner court with apartments or houses on four sides, which suggests the plan of construction of the inner apartments of an Indian house from very ancient times. This plan combined the advantages of seclusion and privacy together with provision for light and air.

Vatsyayana describes with greater fullness the outer chambers which the master called particularly his own and where he spent by far the greater portion of his day and night. An examination of the furniture and equipments of these chambers will give us an insight into the life of the man of wealth and fashion in the third century after Christ. The articles that Vatsyayana first draws attention to, in the master's apartment, are two couches with beds, soft and comfortable and spotlessly white, sinking in the middle, and having rests for the head and feet at the top and the bottom. At the head of his bed is a *kurchasthana*, a stand or perhaps a niche for placing an image of the deity that he worships, as the commentary, 'Jayamangala', explains; besides, at the head there is also an elevated shelf serving the purposes of a table whereon are placed articles necessary for his toilet

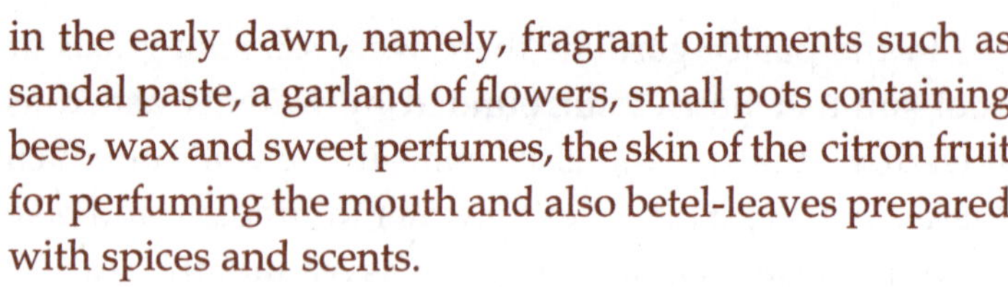

in the early dawn, namely, fragrant ointments such as sandal paste, a garland of flowers, small pots containing bees, wax and sweet perfumes, the skin of the citron fruit for perfuming the mouth and also betel-leaves prepared with spices and scents.

On the floor is a vessel for catching the spittle. On the wall, on brackets (elephants' tusks—*nagadantaka*) are ranged his vina, the national instrument of music in ancient India, a casket containing brushes and other requisites for painting, a book—preferably a poetical work—and garlands of the yellow amaranth (*kurantaka*), chosen because it does not fade or wither soon and therefore is good for decorating the rooms. Not far from the couch, on the floor, is spread a carpet with cushions for the head, and besides, there are boards for playing at chess and dice.

Outside the room is the Nagaraka's aviary where are hung cages of birds for game and sport; we read in the 'Buddhacharita' that the birds in such household aviaries in the city of Kapilavastu were disturbed by the hurried movements of ladies hastening to catch a glimpse of the young prince Siddhartha as he passed along the street. At a somewhat retired spot in the house are places where our Nagaraka amuses himself by working at the lathe or the chisel.

Daily Life of the Nagaraka

Vatsyayana has left us a description of the occupation of the Nagaraka duing the whole of the day, which though brief, yet brings up very beautifully the man of fashion of those days before our eyes. Our Nagaraka gets up early in the morning and after attending to his morning duties and cleaning his mouth and teeth, proceeds to his toilet. The first article in this toilet is the *anulepana,* a fragrant ointment ordinarily made of fine sandalwood paste, or of preparations of a variety of sweet-smelling substances. He applies a suitable quantity of this ointment to his person; it would be considered bad taste if he used too much of this perfume; he then scents his clothes in the sweet-smelling smoke of incense (*dhupa*) thrown into the fire and wears a garland on the head, or hangs it round his neck. He applies collyrium made of various substances to his eyes. To his lips, already reddened by the betel he has chewed, he applies *alaktaka* (a red dye made from lac), to impart a deeper crimson to them and then rubs them over with wax to make the dye fast. Then he looks at himself in a glass, chews spiced betel-leaves to perfume his mouth, and proceeds to attend to his business. He attends to his hair and wears rings on his fingers that are sometimes of great value. He generally wears two garments, a *vasas* or *vastra* and an *uttariya* or a wrap for the upper part of the body.

This upper garment was sometimes very highly scented with rich perfumes or flowers. Bhasa tells us that the rich fragrance of Charudatta's wearing apparel assured Vasantasena that though impoverished, he was not quite unmindful of the amenities of youthful society. At Nanda's house at Kapilavastu when Buddha entered it, some of the maids were preparing the perfumed paste while others were perfuming the clothes. In the 'Lalita-vistara' we read that King Shuddhodana ordered that all those who would attend on Mayadevi on her journey to the garden of Lumbini, should wear clothes, soft and fine, coloured with pleasant dyes and smelling sweet with the best of the scents. Similarly, in another place in the same book, we read of a perfumed garment of the exquisite colour of the *nagakesara*.

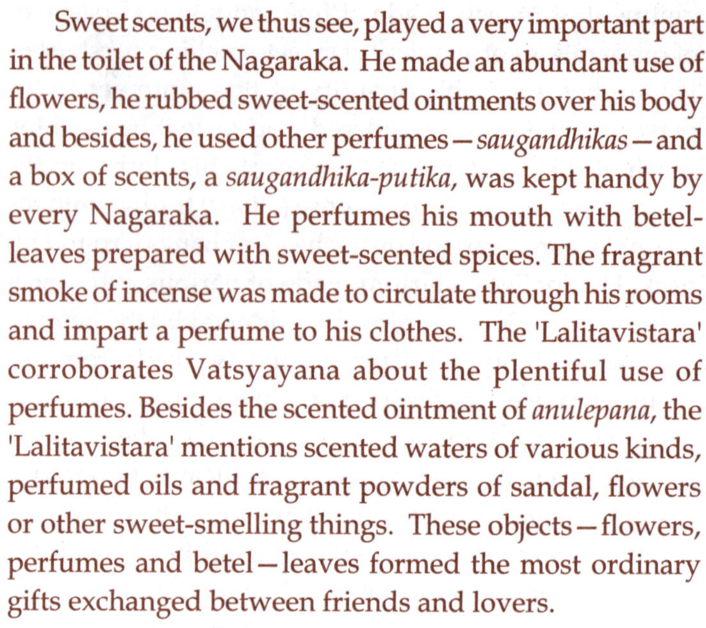

Sweet scents, we thus see, played a very important part in the toilet of the Nagaraka. He made an abundant use of flowers, he rubbed sweet-scented ointments over his body and besides, he used other perfumes – *saugandhikas* – and a box of scents, a *saugandhika-putika,* was kept handy by every Nagaraka. He perfumes his mouth with betel-leaves prepared with sweet-scented spices. The fragrant smoke of incense was made to circulate through his rooms and impart a perfume to his clothes. The 'Lalitavistara' corroborates Vatsyayana about the plentiful use of perfumes. Besides the scented ointment of *anulepana,* the 'Lalitavistara' mentions scented waters of various kinds, perfumed oils and fragrant powders of sandal, flowers or other sweet-smelling things. These objects – flowers, perfumes and betel – leaves formed the most ordinary gifts exchanged between friends and lovers.

After attending to his business in the morning, the Nagaraka takes his bath; this he does every day but there are other attendant circumstances that are repeated at varying intervals. Every other day he gets his limbs massaged and shampooed (*utsadana*); every third day he cleanses his person with soap-like substances that yield a lather with water (*phenaka*). This last was considered an indispensable article for one who aspired to decent life in those days, as we see that even when a man became too poor to maintain himself as a Nagaraka and became a *pithamarda,* his *phenaka* or soap marked him out from ordinary men.

As regards shaving, the Nagaraka was behind the modern man of fashion; he got his chin and lips cleaned every fourth day and this was probably considered conducive to long life, and a more thorough tonsorial operation was performed every fifth or every tenth day.

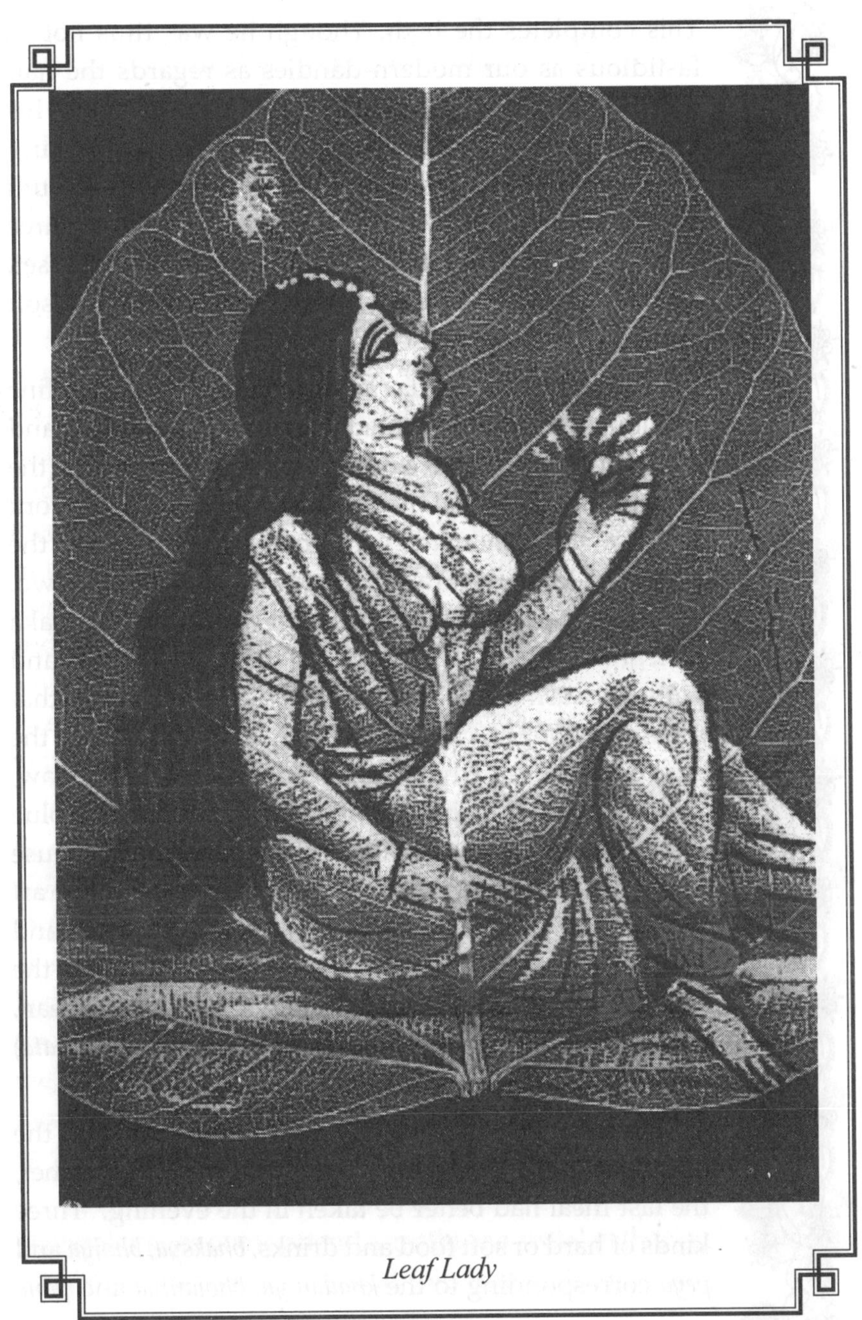

Leaf Lady

intellectural diversions with his friends and in tests of skill in the various arts. At nightfall, our Nagaraka enjoys music, vocal and instrumental ocassionally attended with dances. After music, in his own room which has been made sweet and clean and gay with flowers, and while its fragrant air is charged with the breath of sweet incense circulating through it, the Nagaraka with his associates and friends, awaits there the arrival of his mistress. This completes his daily life.

A word here about the Nagaraka's friends whom we meet again and again in the Kamasutra, will not be out of place. Besides the many artists and craftsmen who served him in his quest of love and pleasure and who are called his *mitras* or companions by Vatsyayana, the Nagaraka appears to have possessed some real, true and devoted friends. Vatsyayana says that fast and genuine friendship often sprang up among those who had grown up together from infancy tended by the same nurse, who in early boyhood were fellow playmates or were at school together, those who were marked by the same temperament and the same tastes in pleasure and sport, were attached to each other by mutual obligations and whose closest secrets were known to each other. Vatsyayana regards it particularly fortunate in friendship when the friendship has come down between two families for several generations, has never been tainted by selfishness or greed, nor has been changed by time or by any considerations whatsoever and where the mutual secrets have never been betrayed.

Sports and Festivities

Besides the various sports and amusements that enlivened the daily life of the Nagaraka, there were many high days and holidays when he made merry with his

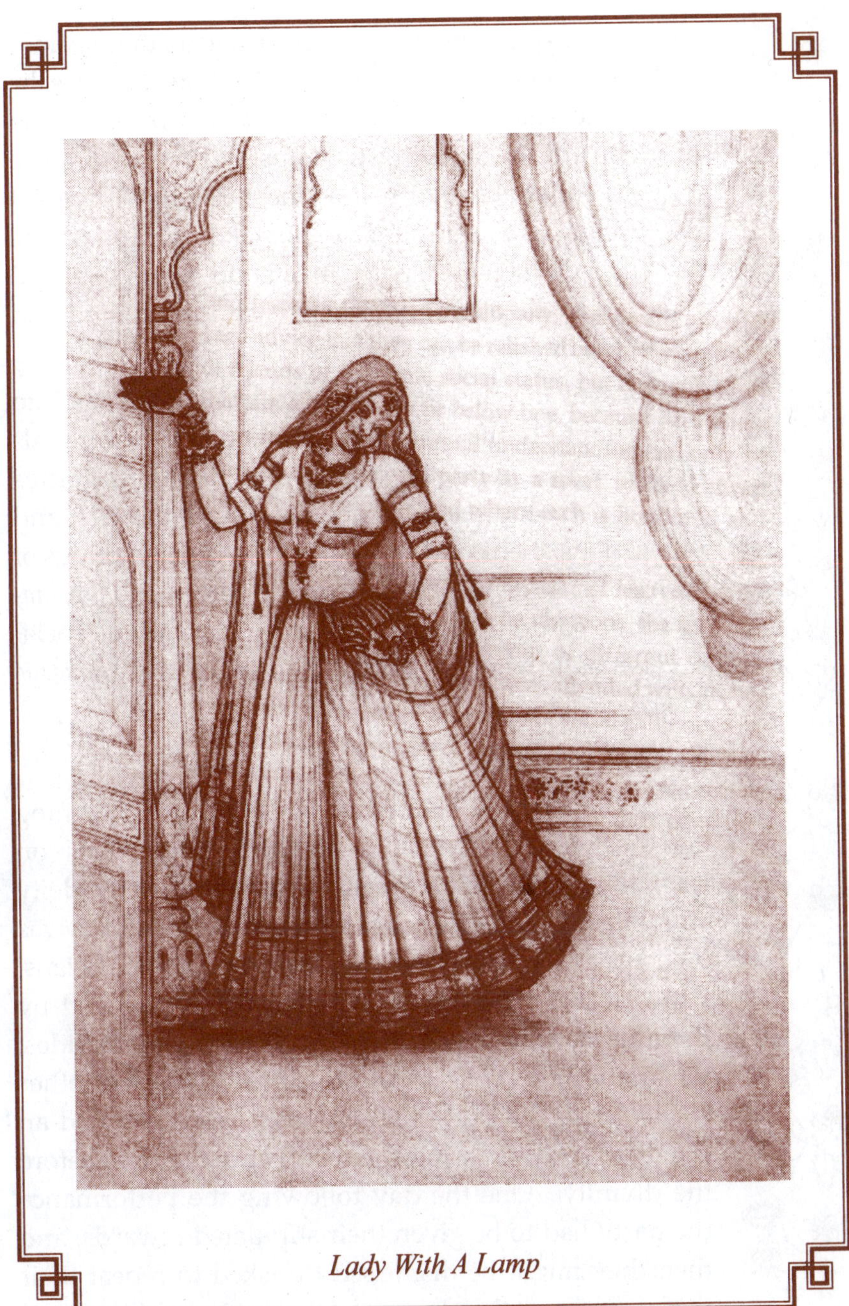

Lady With A Lamp

friends and companions. With regard to all these games and festivities enjoyed in company, Vatsyayana gives the sage advice that they can be relished best in the company of friends of the same social status, but not with those that are either above or below one, because permanent good relations and mutual understanding can only be established when each party in a sport seeks to afford pleasure to the other and where each is honoured and respected by the other.

Vatsyayana classified the occasional festivities into five groups. In the first place he mentions the festivals in connection with the worship of different deities (*samaja*, *yatra* and *ghata*), sometimes attended with grand processions; then come the *gosthis* or social gatherings of both sexes; next *apanakas* or drinking parties and *udyana-yatras* or garden-parties, and last of all, various social diversions in which many persons take part (*samasya-krida*).

Samaja and Gosthi

At the temple of Sarasvati, the goddess of learning and the fine arts, on a fixed day every fortnight, that is on the *tithi* or lunar phase specially auspicious to the deity worshipped, a *samaja* or an assemblage of Nagarakas was held regularly. They were accompanied by musicians, dancers and other artists permanently employed by them for performances in honour of the deity. Besides, when any itinerant parties of actors, dancers or other such "artists" visited the town, they were afforded an opportunity of showing their skill at the temple before the divinity. One the day following the performance the party had to be given their stipulated rewards, and then they might be dismissed or asked to repeat their performances at the pleasure of their patrons. On special occasions, when performances on a grand scale were arranged, parties of actors might co-operate with each other and give a joint performace and it was the duty of the corporation or guild, to which the Nagaraka belonged, to honour and treat with hospitality the strangers who attended these gatherings. Similar festivities of various kinds were held on a grand scale in honour of different deities according to the customs appertaining to each. On some of these occasions there were processions *(yatra)* like the procession of images that Fa-Hien saw in Khotan when "they swept and watered the streets inside the city, making a grand display in the lanes and byways." In these processions both men and women joined and Vatsyayna says that they afforded opportunities for meeting one's lady-love. Even a virtuous matron could attend a religious ceremony with the permission of her husband.

We now come to the *gosthi* or social gathering where the Nagaraka diverts himself in pleasant talk with persons of the same status and position as himself by their education, intelligence, character, wealth and age; that he engages in competitions in making verses or in various other sports of skill and art. Affording, as these *gosthis* did, opportunities for the Nagaraka to exhibit his intellectual accomplishments and mastery of the arts, they were most popular with him, being attended by him every afternoon and they were also held on a comparatively large scale on special occasions.

Of the branches of literary art in which competitions were held, we may glean the following from Vatsyayana's list of the sixty-four arts. There were competitions in the extempore composition of verses, completion of a stanza of which a part only was given, the proper reading of

books with proper intonation and accent, either singly or in groups, the reading of passages in prose or verse that on account of many harsh sounds were hard to pronounce, and the art of composing and expounding passages written in a secret code or cipher. These competitions required knowledge of foreign tongues and provincial dialects, knowledge of lexicons and special vocabularies, of metres and the figures of rhetoric, the knowledge of dramas and their stories, in short, a very comprehensive literary and artistic training. One game is described called *pratimala* in which a number of persons had to recite verses one after another, the condition being that every reciter must repeat a verse commencing with the letter with which the previous speaker's verse ended and any one unable to supply his verse sufficiently quickly had to pay a forfeit.

Besides these literary competitions, there were tests of proficiency in the fine arts such as painting, singing, instrumental music and the like and also of manual skill and dexterity in many of the practical arts such as the stringing together of flowers in a garland and so on.

At these gatherings were invited *ganikas* or brilliant artists who by their education and knowledge of the arts, could please the Nagaraka by meeting him on his own ground, in mental and aesthetic culture, and who were therefore loved and honoured by the people. Sometimes the parties were held at the house of one of the *ganikas*, or the Nagarakas met at each other's house, or they assembled in the *sabha*, the public hall of the city or of the *gana* or corporation to which every citizen belonged. Here the citizens came together to discuss politics and philosophy, or to hold competitions in literature or art, or merely to enjoy themselves in convivial parties. This *sabha* of Vatsyayana is the direct descendant of the *samiti* or *parishad* of the Vedic times, at one of which, that of the Panchalas, Shvetaketu Aruneya, who is reputed to be the founder of the science of erotics, was defeated by a Kshatriya.

At the *gosthis* were also discussed the sixty-four Panchala or kama-kalas and Vatsyayana declares that a person possessing a knowledge of these sixty-four, even though devoid of all the other sciences, leads the talk at the *gosthis* of men and women; and on the other hand, a person who speaks cleverly on other subjects but knows not the sixty-four, is not much respected in the discussions in the assembly of the learned.

At the *gosthi* one is neither to speak too much in Sanskrit for he may then be considered a pedant, just as in England two centuries ago to write English in strict accordance with orthography and syntax was considered not necessary for a gentleman; nor should the Nagaraka speak too much in a local dialect, because then he ran the risk of being regarded as uneducated and uncultured; he should strike a middle course and have full control over both and then he was sure to win great respect. The prevalent language of the period as seen in inscriptions and in the Mahayana literature, bears testimony to the fact that the current speech at the time, at least among the cultured classes, was a mixture of Sanskrit and Prakrit. The learned people like Ashvaghosa, of course, wrote pure Sanskrit, but the language of conversation among the educated was apparently a mixture of Sanskrit and the provincial dialect *(desabhasa)* as recommended by the author of the Kamasutra.

There were *gosthis* for sinister purposes too in the days of Vatsyayana who warns the Nagaraka against frequenting an assembly that is disliked by the people, that is not governed by proper rules and hence is likely to indulge in license or to run beyond the bounds of decency; nor should he attend a *gosthi* that is intent upon doing mischief to others. A person wins success in life by attending an association that makes the imparting of pleasure to people its sole business and has sport and diversion for its sole object.

The *gosthi* on account of its association with art, refinement and culture, was much appreciated by the people in Vatsyayana's times. A Nagaraka was expected to be liberal in spending on *gosthis* and his success in courtship and love depended in no small measure on his power to shine in the sports and festivities including the *gosthi* and *samaja*. In Bhasa's dramas we meet with many references to gosthi; his 'Avimaraka' mourns the supposed loss of his friend who was humorous at *gosthis*.

Women also met together in *gosthis* or social assemblies among themselves. For an unmarried girl it was considered a qualification that she was fond of *gosthis* and *kalas*. Married ladies also sometimes, with the permission of their husbands, instituted among their own friends *gosthis* or social gatherings where they discussed artistic and literary matters. But a married woman who was too fond of instituting *gosthis* was looked upon with suspicion, specially one who arranged such gatherings in the house of a youthful neighbour. In Bhasa's 'Avimaraka' (Act V) the maids invite the Vidusaka to recount a story which they would listen to among their *gosthijanas* in the inner court.

Drinking Parties

Besides the *gosthis* the Nagaraka also met at each

other's house to hold drinking parties where they drank various kinds of liquors with sauces of various tastes and flavours, but abstention from wine was considered a special qualification in a Nagaraka.

Next we come to another diversion which was very dear to the soul of the Nagaraka, *udyana-yatra* or picnics in gardens. Every great city in those days was surrounded by extensive gardens where the resident of the city could find some relief from the congested streets of the town. Around Kapilavastu, says the 'Lalitavistara', five hundred gardens sprang up for the diversions of Bodhisattva, and prince Siddhartha went out through the gates of the city for enjoying himself in the gardens outside. In the Kamasutra also we find that these gardens were outside the town and a whole day was spent in the picnic there. Early in the morning a party of well-dressed Nagarakas would go out of the town mounted on horses accompanied by *ganikas* and followed by servants; there they would arrange for their daily meal and pass the times in pleasant games of chance or in diverting themselves with the fights of cocks, quails or rams or in any other way that they pleased; in the afternoon they would return wearing some token of rememberance of the picnic such as a bunch of flowers or a twig from a garden-tree. Similar parties were enjoyed in connection with sports in water, which took place in artificial lakes or tanks from which all mischievous water-animals had first been removed. Picnicking in the gardens outside the city was very popular in the days of Vatsyayana who again and again speaks of it. His description of *udyana-yatra* agrees in evey particular with that given in 'Mricchakatika', the only difference being that in the drama, Charudatta goes out in a bullock-cart instead of on horseback. A Nagaraka's liberality was often tested by his readiness to spend on these garden picnics and dramatic performances.

A king who has many wives is advised by Vatsyayana to please every one of them by such shows and garden-parties. Unmarried girls, and even married women, sometimes went to these picnics; a virgin on her way to a garden-party was sometimes snatched away from her friends and guardians for the purposes of marriage. Ladies perhaps went on such picnics in parties of their own sex, because Vatsyayana says that *udyan-yatras* afforded opportunities for meeting and making offers of love to them. But picnics arranged by married women appear to be rather rare. It was only a *punarbhu*, that is, a widow who had attached herself to a second husband, that induced her adopted lover to institute these picnics and convivial assemblies at which she herself took part.

Last of all we come to the sports that Vatsyayana calls *samasya-krida* or *sambhuya-krida*, that is, social diversions in which a number of persons took part. He says that they varied with each country and province. Of about a score of them he has given only the names from which their character may sometimes be surmised. Some of them are well-known up to the present day, at least in parts of India, such as Kaumudi-jagara, in which the whole night of the full moon in the month of Ashvina is passed without sleep by playing at dice or similar other amusements, and the Holaka or Holi on the day of the vernal full moon in the month of Phalguna; such is also the Alola-chaturthi or Hindolotsava in the month of Sravana. The Hallisaka, accompanied by dancing and music and supposed to be similar to the Rasotsava described in the 'Bhagavata-Purana,' is referred to by

Vatsyayana and a form of it is still current in Kathiawad. The festival of Suvasantaka reminds us of the Dule-vasamtiya of the Sitabenga Cave-Inscription which tells us that at this "swing-festival of the vernal full-moon, frolic and music abound and people tie around their necks garlands thick with jasmine flowers". We are also reminded of the Kamadevanuyana of Bhasa's Charudatta (Act-I). If appears that persons of both sexes took part in many of these festivities. At such festivals as Kaumudi-jagara, Suvasantaka and Ashtami Chandraka, the women of the cities and towns entered the harem of the king and sported with the royal ladies there.

Sports of Girls

Some of the sports of girls have been described by Vatsyayana, as well as some or their playthings. The girls took delight in making garlands of flowers, building small houses of earth, of wood, playing with dolls, or in cooking imaginary food with such materials as earth, etc. They sometimes played games of chance with dice or cards, or other games like "odd and even," the game of "close fists" and so on; or they might play the game of finding out the middle finger or the sport with six pebbles; sometimes a number of girls played together at games involving some exercise of the limbs such as hide and seek, spinning round holding each other's outstretched arms, blindman's bluff, games with salt or heaps or wheat. We see from this list that many of these sports and games are much the same as those in vogue at the present day among Indian girls and boys.

The games and festivities of the Nagaraka are, as we see from the description given above, the diversions of a seeker after pleasure and amusement – of one that had plenty of leisure to enjoy and an ample fortune to provide the means of enjoyment. Among manly sports, wrestling

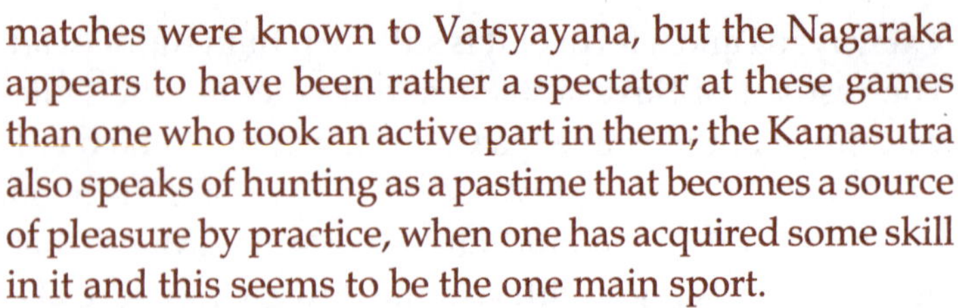

matches were known to Vatsyayana, but the Nagaraka appears to have been rather a spectator at these games than one who took an active part in them; the Kamasutra also speaks of hunting as a pastime that becomes a source of pleasure by practice, when one has acquired some skill in it and this seems to be the one main sport.

We have thus seen that the Nagaraka was a man of considerable intellectual culture and aesthetic refinements, but at the same time he was not very scrupulous with regard to sexual morality. He was the product of an age when wealth and riches were flowing into India through an extensive commerce with the east and the west and the picture that the Kamasutra furnishes of his life also shows the virtues and vices characterstic of such an age. It must not be imagined, however, that the age in which Vatsyayana lived was as a whole an age of gross materialism; it will be a mistake to suppose that the Nagaraka's easy morality was even a main feature of the character of majority of the people. The class which he represents has lived in all ages and in all countries wherever economic prosperity has enabled a section of the people to command and enjoy good things.

We observe that the character of the matron was marked by firmness and purity, modesty and restraint showing that the general ideals of the society had not been lowered since the age of the Dharmasastras. In fact it is apparent from what Vatsyayana says, that the main current of social life had not undergone much transformation and that the ideals set up in Dharma codes still controlled society. He asserts that the whole structure of society is upheld and maintained by the observance of the principle of division of the people into Varnas or classes and into Ashramas or stages of life.

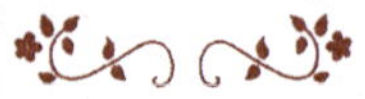

3
The Position of Women

While the life of a Nagaraka has been painted by Vatsyayana as a round of pleasures, that of his wife presents a striking contrast and is a round of duties. The picture presented by him of a wife is in no way inferior to the ideal held up in the Dharmasastras and in many respects he gives greater details. She attends on her husband with all the love and devotion a devotee shows to the deity he worships. She minsters to his personal needs, looks after his food and drink, as well as his toilet and his amusements; she tries to appreciate his likes and dislikes, welcomes his friends with proper presents, respects and loves his parents and relatives and is liberal to his servants; when she finds that he is coming home, she hastens to meet him and waits upon him herself; in his games and sports she follows him; even when offended, she does not speak too bitterly to him.

She may attend a festive assembly only with his permission and in the company of her friends. She does not even give away anything without his knowledge. She should do nothing that might rouse his suspicion against her fidelity; she should avoid the company of women of questionable character such as female ascetics, actresses, fortune-tellers, or women given to the practice of black art, nor should she loiter about in solitary parts of the house. She might take lessons in the Kamasutra or in the subsidiary arts if her husband so wishes, and he may occasionally himself give these lessons. One is here reminded of Bhasa's Udayana who calls his beloved queen "his dear disciple, and of the beautiful line of Kalidasa(with whom our author has so many points of contact) where Aja mourns the loss of Indumati, his "beloved pupil in the fine arts."

There is an atmosphere of control and restraint about her. In her talk she is moderate and never speaks or laughs aloud; she does not return an answer when reproved by her husband's parents. She does not give herself airs when she enjoys great good fortune. In her dress she practices moderation; when going out on festive occasions, she wears a few ornaments and only a few garments of fine and soft texture, uses perfumes and ointments very moderately and adorns herself only with white flowers. But when she is going to meet her husband, she takes the greatest care with her toilet; then she makes herself tidy, sweet and clean, she puts on many ornaments, wears flowers of various hues and smells, uses perfumes and in every way makes herself attractive.

Flowers were worn in garlands hanging from the neck, or in chaplets on the head, or were simply put in the hair., or in elaborate ornaments for the ears (*karnapura* or *karnapatra*). Another item of a woman's toilet was the paint or the dots and patches on the forehead and cheeks, put on in various designs. Sometimes leaves of such plants as *tamala* were used with it, as we find in the 'Saundarananda Kavya'. Vatsyayana advises a wife never to present herself before her husband without some ornaments on her person even when along with him. This idea is found in Indian literature as early as the time of Yaska, who says, "to the man who understands her meaning, the Veda shows herself as a loving wife shows

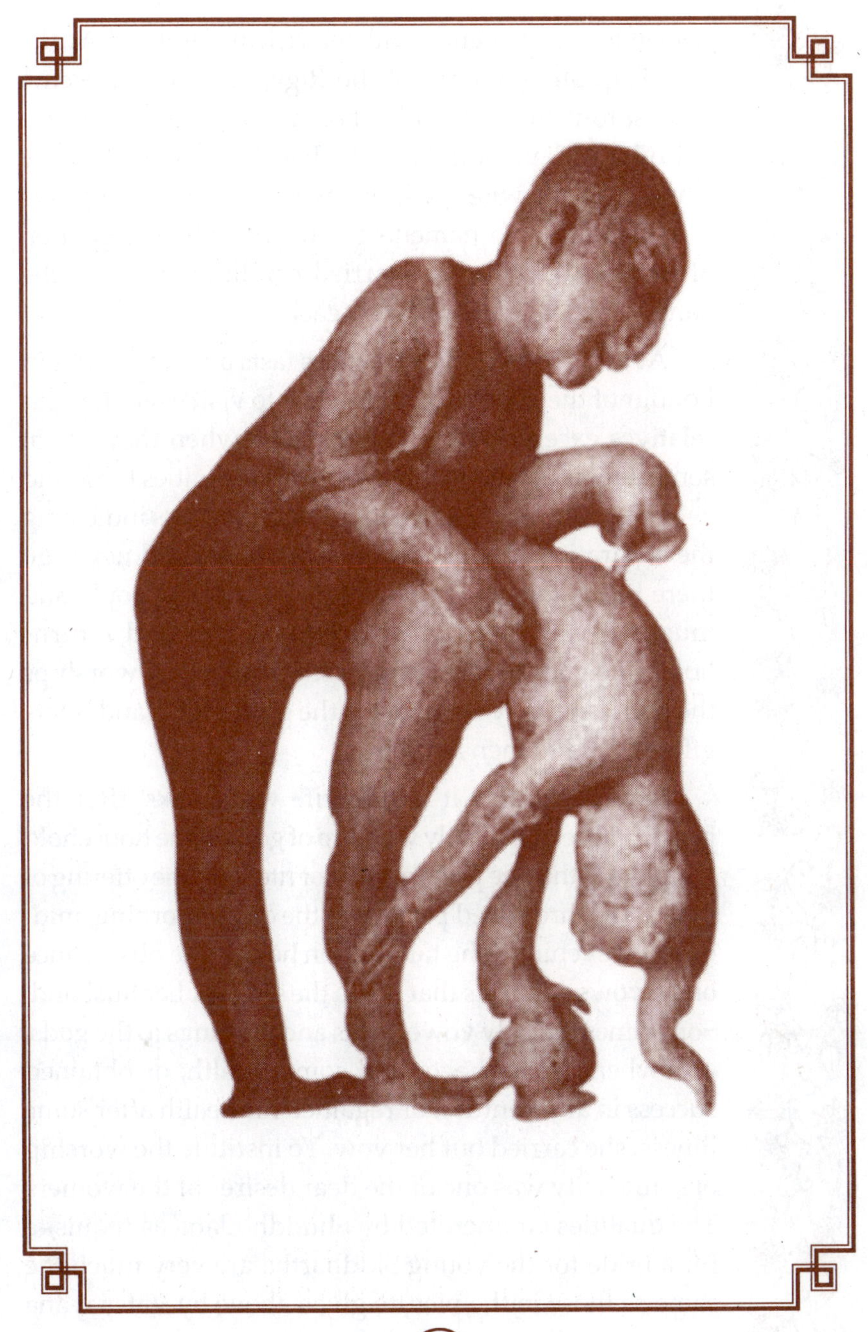

herself to her husband in all her rich apparel. "As Yaska here is quoting a verse of the Rigveda where it occurs at least four times, the idea belongs to the very earliest period of Indian thought. But when the husband is away from home the wife goes, as it were, into mourning; she puts away all her ornaments and finery with the exception of those that mark her married condition, such as the bangles of shells, only one on each wrist.

At that time she also practices fasts and austerities in honour of the gods and does not go to visit even the near relatives except in very urgent cases when they are in some danger, or when there are some festivities there and even then, she must not change her quiet dress indicating the separation (*pravasa-vesha*); and she should never go there but in the company of her husband's people and must not stay there long. When the husband returns home she goes to meet him as she is, then she worships the gods, specially Kamadeva, the god of love, and offers gifts of food to men and birds.

Ordinarily also it is the wife who looks after the performance of the daily worship of gods at the household temple and the due performance of rites and the offering of gifts at the three fixed periods in the day—morning, mid-day and evening. She takes upon herself the observance of the vows and fasts that fall to the share of her husband. Sometimes the lady vowed gifts and offerings to the gods, and when her lord acquired some wealth, or obtained success in any venture, or regained his health after some illness, she carried out her vow. To institute the worship of some deity was one of the dear desires of the women. The qualities enumerated by Shuddhodana as requisite for a bride for the young Siddhartha are very much the same as those in the picture given above by Vatsyayana of a virtuous and devoted wife.

With the permission of her husband the wife takes upon herself the whole care and management of the family. She prepares a budget for the whole year and regulates the expenditure in proportion with the annual income. She must also know how to keep the daily accounts and total up the daily receiptsand expenditure; Manu also lays down that the husband should appoint the wife to receive and spend the wealth, by keeping accounts, as Medhatithi explains. When the husband is inclined to spend beyond his means, or to run into improper expenditure, she remonstrates with him in secret.

She lays in a stock of all articles necessary for consumption and replenished her stores at the proper season,. She knows how to calculate and pay the wages and salaries of the servants, has to look after agriculture and cattle, and also to take care of the animals and birds kept for sport by the master of the house. We have seen that the garden also is a special charge of the lady of the house, When the husband is absent from home she also looks after his affairs and tries to administer them carefully so that they may not suffer by his absence; on such occasions she endeavours to minimize the expenditure to the best of her power and to increase the resources of the family by sales and purchases carried on through trusted servants. She has to attend to the kitchen, and besides, she employs her leisure in spinning cotton and also in doing some weaving.

Poor Women

Many of the poorer women-widows, helpless women,

or those who had adopted the ascetic's vow (*pravrajita*), earned a living by spinning and weaving as at the time of Kautilya, and got their wages from a government officer, the Sutradhyaksha, the Superintendent of Yarn, and the sales and purchases were made with the Panyadhyaksha, the Superintendent of Manufactures. In the villages, the peasant women did various kinds of work under the control of the government officer (Ayuktaka) in charge of the village or the headman who lived upon a share of the agricultural produce. Under his orders these women perform unpaid work for him; they fill up his granaries, take things in or out of his house, clean and decorate his residence, or work in his fields, they also take from him cotton, wool, flax or hemp for spinning yarn and the bark of trees, or thread, for preparing wearing apparel; moreover, they made with him transactions of sale, purchase or exchange of various articles. Similarly, the women in dairy settlements transacted business with the Gavadhyaksa, the Superintendent of Cattle.

The Joint – Family

The joint family system seems to have obtained in Vatsyayana's age. The wife of the householder has to wait upon his parents and to obey them implicitly as we have already seen, and moreover, she has to show proper regard to all senior relations and to his sisters as well as to their husbands. But nowhere are her duties to his brothers mentioned, though a woman with many younger brothers of her husband is referred to in one place showing probably that sometimes the brothers lived together, but more often they established separate households when they got married, as it was prescribed in some of the Dharmasastras; in Manu for example, that after the death of the parents the brothers might live jointly or they might separate for the sake of increasing the dharma, for, if they lived separate, their spiritual merit would increase and hence separation was sanctioned by dharma; the meaning is that if they lived apart "each of them had to kindle the sacred fire, to offer separately the agnihotra, to perform the five great sacrifices and so forth, and hence each gains merit separately." This principle had been recognized from very early times as we have it clearly laid down by Gautama, the author of the earliest of the extant Dharmasutras.

Polygamy

Polygamy appears to have been prevalent in Vatsyayana's days among the wealthy. Kings generally considered it a privilege to have a crowded harem, a harem with a thousand spouses is spoken of by Vatsyayana. This is in line with what the 'Lalita vistara' says about Maya, devi that she was the best and greatest of the thousands of women of Shuddhodana. The 'Buddhacharita' mentions the same fact though not in such extravagant terms. Princes, high officials and the rich also married more than one wife. Vatsyayana says that the wealthy people had generally a plurality of spouses who, outwardly no doubt, appeared to enjoy many objects of pleasure, but in reality, were very miserable indeed, as the husband was but one and the claimants to his affection were many; and he gives the sage advice that it is better to have a poor husband even though he may not have many qualities to recommend him than to have a clever man whose favours have to be shared with many. A single wife for a wealthy man, however, was not unknown: we read in Vatsyayana of a Nagaraka who may be devoted to one wife (*ekacharin*). Prince Nanda of the 'Saundarananda Kavya' was such a person. The majority of the people appeared to have only one wife; but if she had no child, or if she bore only daughters and the continuity of the family was in danger, then the husband might marry again. In case of barrenness, Vatsyayana counsels the wife herself in induce the husband to marry again and look upon the newly married wife as a younger sister. He advises a man with many wives not to be partial, neither to show any disregard towards any one in particular, nor to allow any offence on the part of any one of them to pass unnoticed.

Antahpura

We have already seen that every house had an *antahpura*, or inner suite of apartments where the ladies resided in seclusion, guarded against intrusion from any stranger; not even women except those of approved character, were admitted within. Bhasa's Vasantasena complains that she had the misfortune of not being entitled to enter into the inner courtyard of Charudatta's house. It was not considered decent for the wife of a Nagaraka to stand at the door and look out or to observe people in the street from her windows; even when she hastens to meet her husband coming home, she does not go out into the street or to the door but waits for him inside the house. Nevertheless, on the occasion of religious festivities and processions, she could accompany the images of the gods with the permission of her husband. The inability of women to protect themselves against temptations as compared with men, is recognized by Vatsyayana and he like Manu, condemns the absence of a restraining guardian for a woman.

The kings having a large number of wives took greater care than the ordinary Nagaraka in confining them in seraglios gurarded by officers of proved honesty and purity. No man was allowed to enter into the royal harem except relatives and servants and in some provinces, artisans; Brahmanas were allowed to get into the harem for supplying flowers to the ladies, with whom they conversed separated by a screen. There were in the harem female officers, the *kanchukiya* and the *mahattarika,* who carried presents of garlands, perfumes and garments from the ladies to the king who also sent gifts in return. In the afternoon, the king paid a visit to the harem and met all the ladies assembled together and conversed with them in accordance with their rank and position.

Education of Women

The fact that the mistress of the house was expected to keep the daily accounts, to prepare the annual budget of receipts and expenditure, and supervise in general over the purse, proves, beyond a doubt, that women ordinarily were literate. Besides, from what Vatsyayana says, it is apparent that an ordinary woman could receive and reply to love letters smuggled into ear ornaments, chaplets or garlands made of flowers carried by female messengers (*patrahariduti*). Such love letters not infrequently, contained verses and songs having special reference to the beloved and replies were obtained from her. Unless women had some education, this would be without meaning.

Higher education (*sastragrahana*), however, was not so commen among them, as. Vatsyayana himself says that women did not ordinarily get any education in the sastras, but our author avers that the daughters of kings and nobles, as also the *ganikas*, were highly educated and had their intelligence trained and sharpened by the sastras, and he advises that a woman might learn either the whole or a part of the work *(sastra)* composed by himself from a person who by character and attainments could be trusted. The sixty-four subsidiary sciences that had to be studied along with the Kamasutra, included many that required, as we have seen, no inconsiderable proficiency in belles lettres, in the humanities in general.

Such accomplishments as extempore composition of verses (*manasi-kavyakriya*) and the completion of fragmentary verses (*kavya-samasyapuranam*) required a ready facility in versification that could be acquired only by a highly educated girl. And such sports as *pratimala* required the memorizing of a large mass of verses and good literature. In Vatsyayana's opinion a knowledge of the Kamasutra with its subsidiary sciences would be useful to all women, both high and low, rich and poor. A poor woman who on account of the absence of her husband, finds herself in great distress and difficulty, might earn a decent living even in a foreign country by means of the knowledge of these sciences.

A woman whose husband has been away from home without making provision for her, is advised by Manu also to live by the arts, by such *silpas* as have nothing reprehensible in them. On the other hand, Vatsyayana affirms that a daughter of wealthy parents, if accomplished in the arts, might win the affection of her husband even if he happens to have a large number of wives. We see, moreover, from Vatsyayana's work, as well as from contemporary literature, that a knowledge of the arts was considered necessary for all women. The bride for prince Siddhartha was required, according to his father, to be versed in the sacred literature *(sastra)* and skilled in the arts, even like a *ganika*. The *dharama-buddha* could be born only of a mother versed in many sciences, and Mayadevi satisfied this requirement, besides, she was well skilled in the arts.

Widow Remarriage

The position of a widow who wished for a second husband, has been clearly defined by Vatsyayana. There was no regular marriage for a widow; but if a woman who had lost her husband, was of weak character and was unable to restrain her desires, she might ally herself for a second time to a man who was a seeker after pleasures (*bhogin*) and was desirable on account of his excellent qualities as a lover, and such a woman was called a *punarbhu* Vatsyayana quotes the opinion of several teachers as to how far, in the selection of her second master, the *punarbhu*. should be swayed by the excellence of the qualities of the man of her choice or by the chances of participating in the joys of life, and he concludes that in his opinion it was best for her to follow the natural inclinations of her own heart. The connection with her was of a loose character and she enjoyed a degree of independence unknown to the wife wedded according to sacramental rites.

When the *punarbhu* seeks her lover's house, she assumes the role of a mistress, he patronises his wives, is generous to his servants and treats his friends with familiarity; she chides the lover herself if he gives any causes for quarrel. She shows greater knowledge of the arts than his wedded wives and seeks to please the lover with the sixty-four kamakalas. She takes part in sports and festivities, drinking parties, garden-picnics, and other games and amusements. She might leave her lover (*nayaka*), but if she did so of her own accord, she had to restore to him all presents given by him, except the tokens of love mutually exchanged between them; if she is driven out, she does not give back anything.

The position of the *punarbhu* is therefore quite distinct from that of the wedded wife who participated with her husband in all religious observances and had to live with decency in the *antahpura*; the position of the *punarbhu* approaches nearer to that of a mistress than that of a wedded wife. In the king's harem where there were separate quarters and suites of chambers for the various types of women, the *punarbhus* occupied a position mid-way between the devis or queens who were quartered in the innermost apartments, and the *ganikas* and actresses in the outermost, and this exactly indicates also the position occupied by them in society.

Vatsyayana indicates this in another place where he places the *punarbhu* between the virgin (*kanya*) and the courtesan (*veshya*) and says that the establishment of sexual relations with either the courtesans or the *punarbhus* was not considered as right, neither was it absolutely condemned, because pleasure was the guiding motive in all such connections. It is clear that in Vatsyayana's opinion there could not be any second marriage of the widow. Manu, whose code must have received its present form about that time, declares in unmistakable terms that in the sacred texts concerning marriage, the remarriage of widows, the question of widow-remarriage shows that in his days public opinion

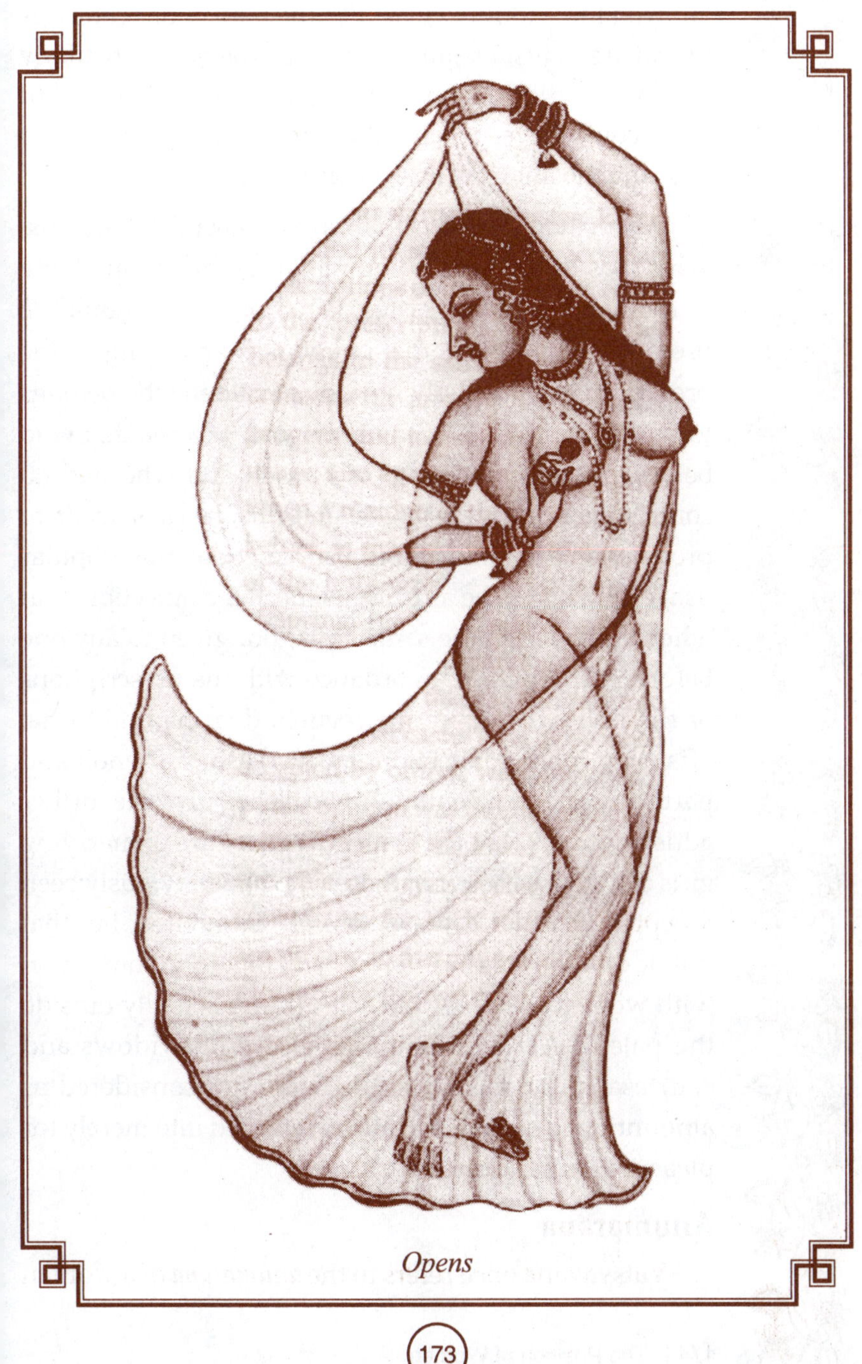

Opens

allowed the widow to live with the man of her choice as his mistress, just as public opinion was not particularly nice or fastidious about making love to courtesans, but they could never receive the same regard, nor acquire the same position, as the married wife.

About the question of marriage in general, Vatsyayana gives it as his considered opinion that for a man of any of the four varnas or castes, kama or desire should be provided its scope in the acceptance, according to the prescriptions of the holy writ, of a maiden who belongs to the prescriptions of the holy writ, of a maiden who belongs to the same caste as himself and who had no contact with any one before, and this, he says, leads to progeny and to fame and is also sanctioned by popular usage; and again, he affirms, in another connection, that when a maiden of the same caste, not given to any one before, is married in accordance with the prescriptions of the holy writ, then one secures dharma and artha, offspring, high connection, an increase of friends and partisans, and also genuine, untarnished love. He further adds definitely that the contrary procedure of marrying girls of higher castes or of those who had previously been accepted by others, was absolutely prohibited, but that public opinion was indifferent with regard to connection with women of the lower castes (if not actually outside the pale of Aryan society), as also with widows and courtesans, for such relations were not considered as amounting to marriage at all, but entered into merely for pleasure for its own sake.

Anumarana

Vatsyayana once refers to the *anumarana* of a woman

upon the death of her lover; perhaps it has a reference to the practice of *sahamarana* or dying with the husband, that is,burning herself on the same funeral pyre, but we cannot be sure about it upon such meager evidence.

Female Ascetics

Some women also took the monastic vow like men and lived upon the charity of the people. Nuns of the three main religions of India at that time are referred to in the Kamasutra. We have the Buddhist nun *shramani*, and her Jain sister, *ksapana* or *ksapanika;* and associated with them we find the *tapasi* whom I take to be the woman who belonging to the Brahmanic faith, has renounced the world. Besides, we read of women who had their heads shaven (*mundah*). All of them are generally spoken of as *pravrajitas* or *bhiksukis,* i.e., female ascetics or mendicants. It appears, from what Vatsyayana says, that these female mendicant orders did not enjoy a high reputation for morality: they are included among those who are declared to be company unfit for decent married ladies.

Some of the mendicant women were proficient in the arts and their help was often sought by the Nagaraka in affairs of love; the house of the *bhiksuki* often formed the rendezvous for lovers; she was often employed to carry messges of love and was regarded as a go-between who could easily create confidence and succeed in her mission. Vatsyayana, however, positively asserts that the love of the female ascetic was never to be sought for by a Nagaraka, though a former teacher had expressed a contrary view.

All this does not imply that female ascetics were in general considered as depraved but that some of them

abused the confidence of the public and thus forfeited the respect to which they had previously been regarded, just like some of the male ascetics and mendicants who erred from the right path, and we learn form Kautilya that the respect which the *parivrajika* or *bhiksuki* commanded in society was made use of in order to fish out political secrets. In Bhavabhuti's 'Malatimadhava' we find the *parivrajika*, Kamandaki, represented as a highly respectable lady who took great interest in the love affair between the hero and the heroine and worked hard for its fruition. This drama is an illustration, as it were, of the Kamasutra, and Bhavabhuti in this drama shows himself very well-versed in Vatsyayana's writings.

The Postion of the Ganikas

In the age of Vatsyayana, the ganika, or the educated and accomplished woman about the town, occupied a peculiar postion. Though belonging to the class of "public women", still she appears to have been treated with special consideration. But it was not every courtesan that received this appellation: it was only when a woman of this class was marked out by high intellectual attainments, and striking pre-eminence in the arts that she won the coveted title of ganika. She must have her mind cultivated and trained by a thorough education (*sastra-prahatabuddhih*) and Vatsyayana lays down that it is only when a courtesan is versed in both the series of sixty-four arts or *kalas* enumerated by him and is endowed with an amiable disposition, personal charms and other winning qualities, that she acquires the designation of a ganika and receives a seat of honour in the assemblies of men.

She is always honoured by the king and is highly

lauded by men qualified to appreciate merit; her favours and company are sought for, and she becomes in fact, the observed of all observers, a model and pattern for all. In the 'Lalitavistara', king Shuddhodana desires for the young Siddhartha a bride who was as much learned in the sastras and as accomplished in the arts as a ganika. 'Bharata's 'Natyasastra', which is a work of the same period, speaks equally, if not more enthusiastically, about the excellences of the ganika. Bharata describes her as one who knows the practical application of various arts, who possesses deep knowledge of many of the sciences *(sastras)*, who is skilled in the sixty-four *kalas* and in dancing to the accompaniment of music, whose conduct is marked by respect towards superiors, by graceful and engaging manners, by charming gestures and sweet blandishments; who possessed strength and firmess of mind and at the same time modesty and a sweetness of temper; who is free form the characteristic defect of women; who speaks gracefully and clearly; who is clever in work and does not get tired; a woman possessed of all these rare qualities and accomplishments would be called a ganika.

That she was regarded by Bharata as a woman of great education and culture appears from the fact that the ganika, when introduced as a character in a drama, is, according to him, to speak Sanskrit. The uses to which the ganika puts her money are also characterized by a desire for public good and her charity shows the noble tendencies of her cultured mind. The ganikas of the highest class, says Vatsyayana, consider it as the highest gain to themselves when they receive sufficient money to spend on the building of temples, excavation of tanks, planting of gardens, erection of bridges and of homes for sacrifice and ceremonies or the institution of permanent arrangements for the worship of the gods. They valued very highly the chance of giving away cows to Brahmanas, of course through a third person, because no Brahmana would accept anything from a courtesan.

The ganika literally appears to mean a woman who is the member of a *gana* or corporation, whose charms are the common poetry of the whole body of men associated together by a common bond, economic or political. Manu associates the ganika in one verse saying that the food offered by both were equally to be refused by a Brahmana. The *gana* might be a corporation of citizens, the *nagarika jana-samavaya* of Vatsyayana, like the one to which our Nagaraka belonged, or it might be a political body like that of the Licchavis of Vaishali whose ganika, Ambapalika, was a glory of their capital and was credited with all the virtues and qualities contemplaed by Vatsyayana and Bharata, thus testifying that their definitions were not fanciful and imaginary. We read in the 'Mahavagga' that she was charming, attractive, graceful, possessed of a fine and tender complexion, generous and proficient in dancing, song and music.

The wealth and power that the ganika of Vaisali possessed and the position that she occupied, were in no way inferior to those of the best of the proud Licchavis; her train was as numerous and as sumptuously decorated, her carriages were as magnificent as those of the Licchavis against whom she drove up axle to axle, wheel to wheel, and yoke to yoke. Her presence made the city of Vaisali shine forth in great splendour and glory. She constituted, as it were, a valued institution of the city, the high model

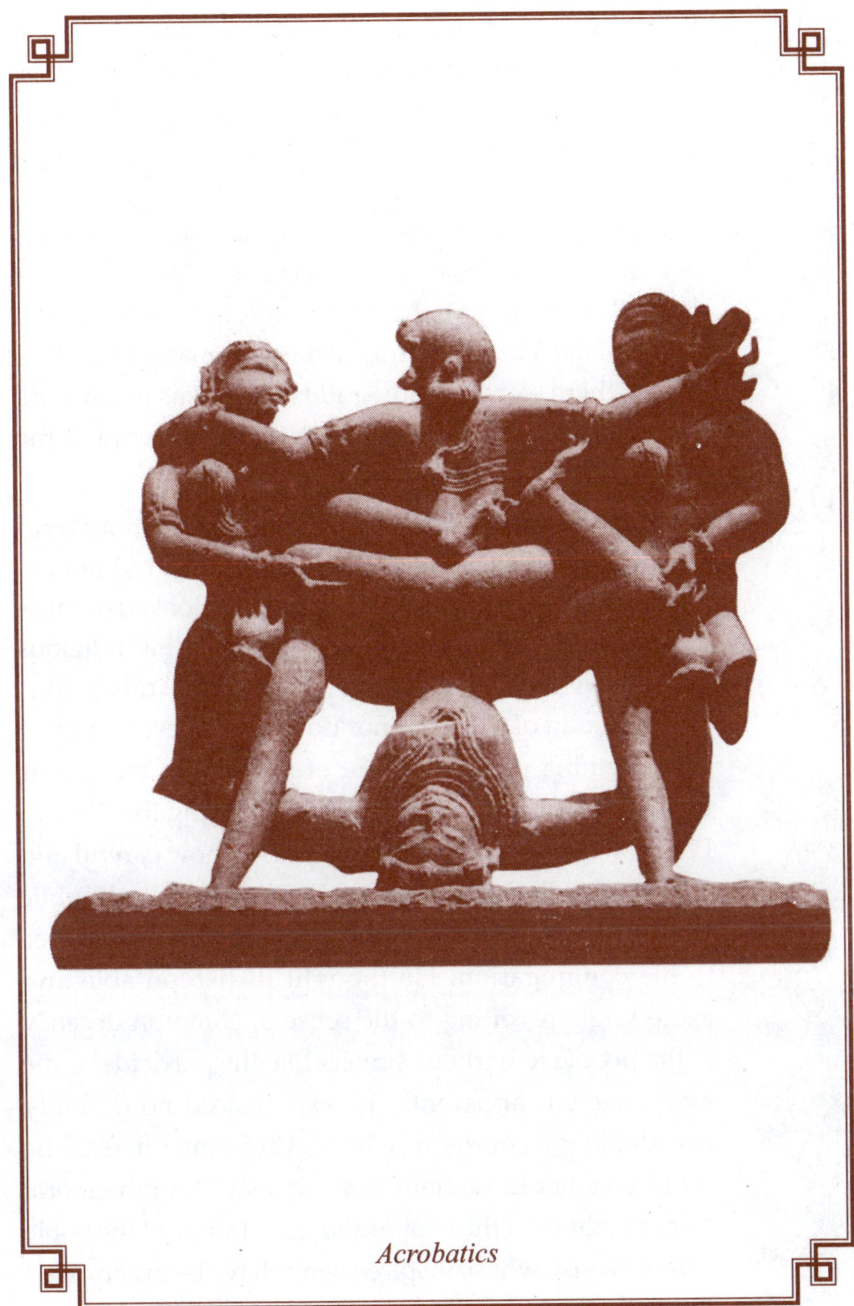

Acrobatics

of beauty and art thus set up by the ganika of Veshali roused a merchant of the rival city of Rajagaha to induce king Bimbisara to have this institution of ganika in his own capital which suffered in this respect in comparison with the chief city of the *ganarajya* or republic of the Licchavis. It shows that in those early times ganikas were not so numerous as they became in Vatsyayana's days. But we observe that in the days of Katyayana, the author of the 'Varttika Sutras' of the grammatical school of Panini, there were already guilds of ganikas *(ganikyam)*, as explained in the '*Mahabhasya*', just as we read of the *ganika sangha* in Vatsyayana.

We may also note the fact that Buddha excludes from his fold the eunuch and the hermaphrodite, but not the ganika, who does not appear to have been looked upon as a moral outcaste past redemption. The Buddhist religious books have hardly anyting to say against Ambapalika, the courtesan of Vaishali, nor do they suggest that there was anything peculiar or out of the way in the favour that Buddha showed towards her. Reading the 'Vinaya Pitaka' we are indeed astonished to see how careful and anxious the Buddha was in order not to offend public opinion and to give a decent and respectable appearance to his congregation. He thought it disreputable and exceedingly revolting to the sense of common decency of the people to harbour sinners like the parricide or the matricide, but apparently he experienced no diffculty in ordaining a courtesan who had reformed herself; he could take her in without causing a shock to the moral susceptibilities of the people and in fact some of the noble sisters (*theris*), whose inspired songs have been compiled in the Therigatha, and reformed their life which before ordination was not quite above reproach.

The position that the ganika enjoyed may be explained by the fact that in a society characterized by aesthetic refinement as was that of the age of Vatsyayana, women who possessed special proficiency in the arts were respected for the value of their art, and their company was sought for by all lovers of art for long training; and education needed for the acquisition of such literary and artistic accomplishments as the ganika possessed, could not be obtained by a girl who was married and had to manage a household, expecially as she was married rather early, though Vatsyayana's chapter on courtship shows that many of them remained unmarried even after puberty.

Moreover, it was certainly not considered decent for such a girl to attend the public schools of arts or *gandharva shalas,* where the daughters of the ganikas received lessons in the arts, and formed, as Vatsyayana says, acquaintance with the sons of the wealthy citizens, nor could any but very wealthy parents afford to give their daughters such education at home. Where the parents were very rich, as in the case of the daughters of princes and high offcials, they did receive, as we have seen before, a thorough education in the arts and sciences.Gopa was as learned and clever as any ganika, as the 'Lalitavistara' says. Then again, the wedded wife, on account of her manifold duties in the household, could not cultivate the arts as thoroughly as she would like to; besides, the great regard for purity in the married woman and the strict and rigid rules that guided her conduct even in the age of Vatsyayana, prohibited, as we have seen above, her receiving lessons in the arts except from her own husband.

We see, therefore, that the ganikas, like the hetaerae in the Athens of Pericles, were generally more educated and better skilled in the arts than the married women, and the Nagarakas, though they had devoted wives at home, as the ideal of a wife drawn by Vatsyayana shows, were attracted by the intellectual and artistic qualities of the educated ganika. Such a noble soul as Bhasa's Charudatta, though he had a devoted wife at home, who was ready to sacrifice the last bit of her personal property for his sake and for whom he himself had a great regard, had no scruple in falling in love with the actress Vasantasena and the 'Mricchakatika' makes him even marry her. With such ideals the devoted wife as we have in Vatsyayana and in Bhasa's Charudatta, it cannot be said with any sound reason that the Nagaraka sought the company of the ganika because his home was miserable or unbearable, but evidently he was drawn by her accomplishments. Even the general public, though they despised her for the life she led, tolerated her on account of her high artistic qualifications which they found on many occasions to enjoy and appreciate at the *preksanakas* or performances at the festive assemblies (*samajas*) such as we have described above.

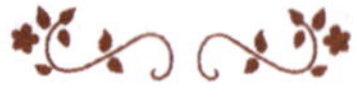

4
The Arts in Those Times

The age of Vatsyayana being characterized by very refined tastes and aesthetic perceptions, as we have seen above, there was joy and consequently beauty in life, and it was necessarily an age when the arts flourished and the crafts prospered. Vatsyayana's Nagaraka is a man of varied culture and from the picture that we have obtained of his life and surrounding, of his home and friends, and of his sports and amusements, there can be no doubt that he was a great patron of the arts; in fact, it is evident that every one who aspired to be a member of cultured society, had to acquire some proficiency in poetry and music, painting and sculpture and to possess some knowledge of a host of minor arts, the sixty-four *kalas* enumerated by our author.

This knowledge of the arts was evidently an essential part of his education and without this modicum of practical acquaintance with them he would not be respected, as Vatsyayana says, in the assemblies of the cultured and educated people. The ideal Nagaraka, according to Vatsyayana, was he who possessed, in addition to a healthy physique, good birth and independent means of livelihood, a knowledge of the various arts, who was learned and eloquent and was, moreover, a poet, well skilled in telling stories, who was fond of all the literary and artistic competitions and festivities including *gosthis* and dramatic performances and, above all, a person whose character was marked by largeness of heart and liberality, by affection and love.

Skill in the sixty-four arts subsidiary to the Kamasutra as well as a knowledge of the sutras themselves was an essential part of the qualification of every cultured man and woman. To win a girl in marriage called for an exercise of many of the arts. A maiden had to be propitiated by rare and curious objects of art, by nicely recited romances and by sweet songs; if she showed a partiality for feats of magic, her favour was to be won by performing various tricks of legerdemain if she manifested a curiosity for the arts, her lover must demonstrate before her his skill in them; the art of gathering flowers in bouquets, or weaving them into chaplets and garlands was specially to be cultivated. Tournaments in which a charming and rarely accomplished girl like Gopa was the prize of the victor (*jaya-pataka*), appear to have been held in cities ruled by a semirepublican government like that of the Sakyakula.

If a man was uncultured and ignorant of the arts it would be a source of great sorrow to his wife who, Vatsyayana suggests, might herself be more proficient in them than he. In the 'Lalitavistara' we find that unless Siddhartha showed his skill in some of the arts (*silpas*), Dandapani Sakya refused to give his girl in marriage to him, prince though he was. It may easily be imagined that art in all its forms was likely to develop and prosper in a society where men and women were inspired by such ideals, and that at the same time the sciences that analysed and ministered to the manifold forms of artistic expression of this highly intellectual and cultured community also grew and were assiduously pursued.

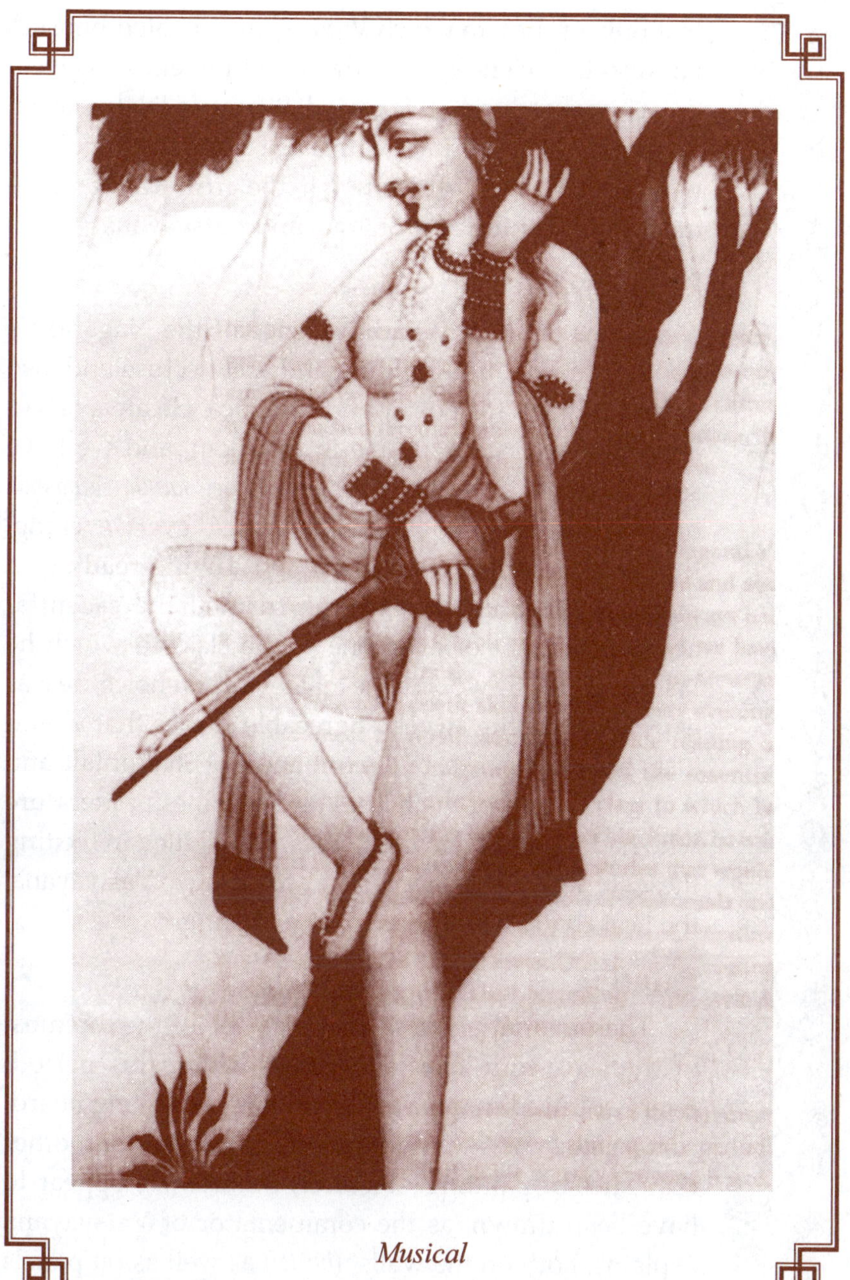

Musical

Not only erotics, to which Vatsyayana devoted himself, but also the sciences of aesthetics and poetics receive a great impetus during this period. Bharata's 'Natyasastra' appears to be a product of this age of aesthetic culture which reached its culmination in the great Kalidasa, the most careful student of Bharata and Vatsyayana.

Literary Art

We have already had evidence of the Nagaraka's good taste in house-building and architecture and also of his fondness for poetry and romance. He always had a poetical work on a table in his room, and we have seen from his skill at the *gosthis* where *kavya-samasyas* or competitions in poetic skill were held every evening, that readiness in versification and a wide reading of poetical literature in general, formed the essential accomplishment of everyone of the class to which he belonged. While wooing the maiden of his choice, he was expected to recite sweetly agreeable stories that would just apply to his case, or the romances of Shakuntala and Avimaraka and of the heroes and heroines of literature who had prospered in their loves. One skilled in reciting these stories and romances had, according to Vatsyayana, the best chance of success in love-making.

Painting

The pictorial art, *alekhyam,* was one of the foremost of the sixty-four *kalas* cultivated during this period. Every cultured man had in his house a drawing board, *citraphalaka,* and a vessel for holding brushes and other requisites of painting. Pictures, *chitrakarma,* appear to have been drawn, as the commentator of Vatsyayana explains, both on the walls (*bhitti*) as well as on panels or boards (*phalaka*); Vatsyayana advises a lover who wants to attract the attention of the lady whose charms have captivated him, to put in places frequented by her, paintings (probably representing himself) done on panels; in another place we read of a kiss imprinted on a picture *(chitrakarma),* most probably on a wall. For *chitrakarma* or painting, the surface of the wall appears to have been most ordinarily used in ancient India, as appears from a passage in the 'Mudraraksasa' where the futility of the earnest efforts of a statesman is compared to the composition of a picture without the wall. The same idea is found in the 'Lalitavistara' where the daughters of Mara declare that it was easier to paint pictures on the sky than to tempt Bodhisattva. Bharata clearly refers to fresco-painting by the phrase *chitrakarma;* he says that the walls of the theatre-hall were to be decorated with *chitrakarma* after they had been carefully plastered, coated with lime and nicely polished, the paintings consisting of the representation of great deeds. It is fortunate that in our country where we have so few pictorial records of the past, the caves at Ajanta have preserved a few frescoes, the solitary survivals of this age of prolific artistic production.

Vatsyayana speaks also of the *akhyanaka-pata* which is evidently a roll of canvas containing the representation of short story in several scenes like the *yamapata* which was spread by a spy of Chanakya before the people in Chandanadas's house and was exhibited by him with songs; we may add that the direct descendant of this *yamapata* may still be seen in the villages of Bengal. Balls with various designs painted on them in a variety of colours, as also water jugs of various elegant shapes with may paintings, are mentioned by Vatsyayana as welcome

presents to a maiden whose favours one is counting. The 'Lalitavistara' mentions a similar plaything for children, jugs beautifully painted on the outside but containing valueless things within.

According to Vatsyayana, a welcome object of presentation to maidens was a colour-box (*patolika*) containing the following course:-- *alaktaka* (the red dye obtained from lac), *manahsila* (red arsenic), *haritala* (yellow orpiment), *hingula* (vermillion) and *shyamavarnaka;* the last named appears to be a vegetable dye, black, blue or green because the word *shyama* is used to signify all these colours. The commentator says that it means a powder used in painting, or *rajavarta*, a mineral substance. A painter surrounded by many cups (*mallakas*) of wet colours is referred to in Bhasa's Charudatta. Jayamngala quotes a beautiful verse apparently from *shilpasastra* about the six great requisites of painting, "knowledge of appearances, correct perception, measure and structure of forms, action of feelings on forms, infusion of grace or artistic representation, similitude and artistic manner of using the brush and colours. "Bharata speaks of the pictorial representation of the feelings or other sentiments, the *rasas,* by different colours, the erotic or amatory sentiment is represented by the *shyama* or dark colour spoken of above, the sentiment of mirth by white; the piteous sentimentis grey (*kapota*) and the choleric is red the heroic is yellowish white (*gaura*) and the terrible, black, the repulsive is blue and the amazing, yellow.

Sculpture

Sculpture flourished as much as painting in the age of Vatsyayana as is fully borne out by the numerous sculptural records that have come down to our time

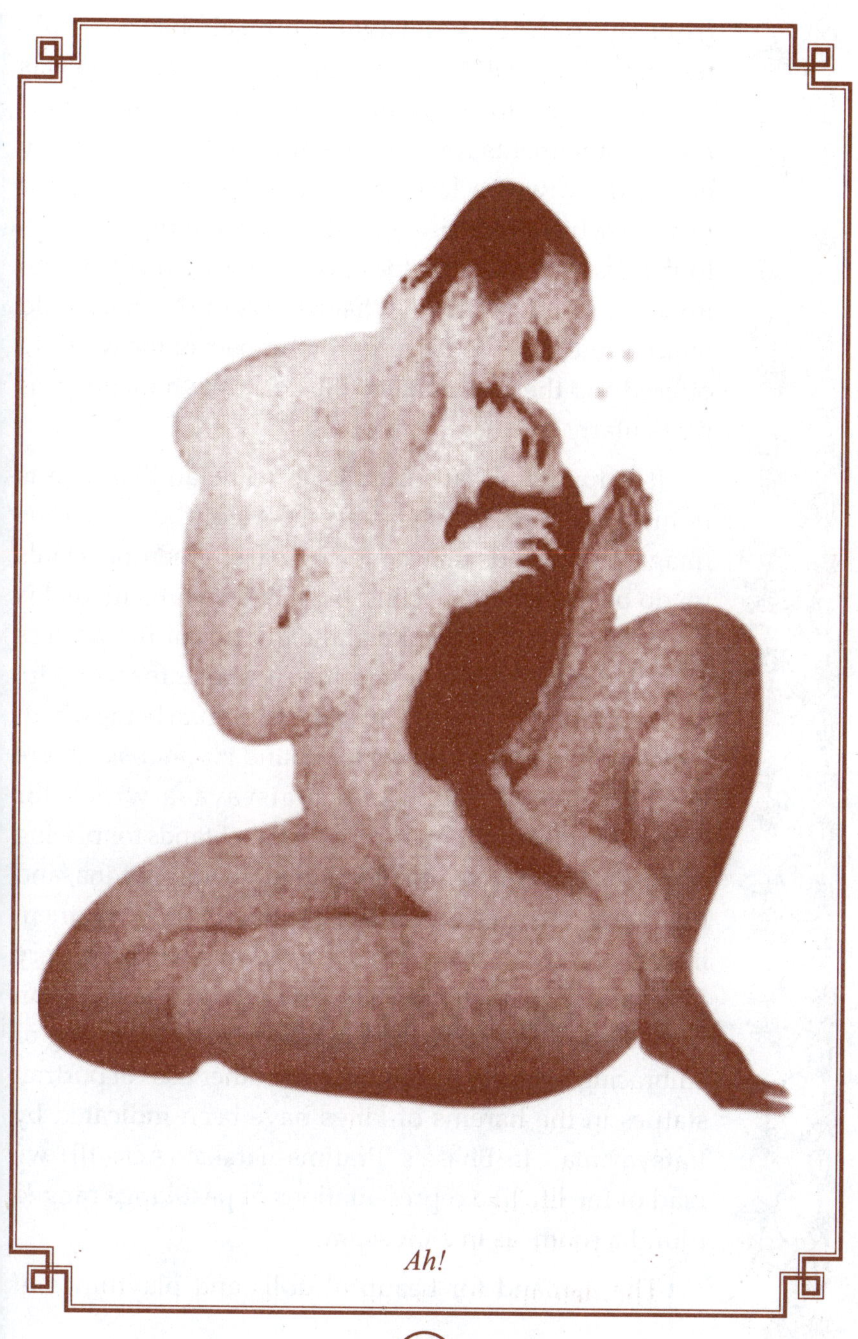

Ah!

from the period. Vatsyayana himself bears ample testimony to it: *takshana,* carving on wood or stone was one of the sixty-four arts and every Nagaraka had in his house implements for working at it; similarly, in every house there was a lathe and other arrangements for turning which, likewise, had its place among the sixty-four *kalas*. Vatsyayana does not expressly mention an image of a god, but from what he says of the household temple where the gods were worshipped, of the worship offered and the gifts made to the deity to whom one was particularly devoted.

It is apparent that such images were familiar objects in his days. The 'Lalitavistara' speaks of the numerous images of the gods that came down from their pedestals to do obeisance to the child Buddha when he made his appearance in the Devakula, the quarter of the palaces occupied by the gods. Besides these images for worship, representations in wood and stone of human beings, both male and female-*purushapratima* and *stripratima*—were used by the class for whom Vatsyayana wrote, for decoration and as appertenances of love. Stands for placing images, or *pindolikas,* are mentioned by Vatsyayana, and life-size statues in wood or stone evidently stood on them in every Nagaraka's house, as Vatsyayana speaks of very familiar uses made of them by lovers who often gave an indication of their passion for a lady by slyly kissing or embracing a statue her sight. Similar other uses of portrait statues in the harems of kings have been indicated by Vatsyayana. In Bhasa's 'Pratima-nataka' (Act -III) we read of the life like representations of past kings ranged round a room as in a museum.

The demand for beautiful dolls and playthings of

which the girls in Vatsyayana's age appear to have been very fond, offered a vast field for the exercise of the plastic art. Vatsyayana advises a young man trying to win the affection of a maiden to present her with dolls made of wood, horn, ivory, cloth, wax, plaster or earth. Erotic pairs of human figures made of wood might also be presented; such erotic pairs (*mithunam*) cut of the leaves of trees were also sent by sweethearts to each other. Playthings liked by girls are miniature cooking utensils, small temples of the gods *(devakula-grihaka),* toy animals like goats or rams and playthings made of earth, split bamboo or wood, such as cages of birds, small vinas, stands for images, ear ornaments made of wax or whatever other objects of art might be demanded by the girl of his choice, must be presented by the man courting her either openly or in secret.

Music

Three *kalas* appertaining to music, singing (*gita*), playing on instrument (*vadya*) and dancing (*nritya*) have been given by our author the first place in the list of arts; besides, there are more—*udakavadya* or playing on cups filled with water in varying proportions and *vina, damaruka-vadyani,* that is, playing on string instruments of which the chief was the *vina* and also on percussion instruments represented by the *damaru*. This last most probably represents the earliest from which in course of time had evolved the *mridanga,* which has lately been proved by one of our eminent scientists to be the most scientifically constructed percussion instrument ever used. The *mridanga* was already known to the 'Mahavagga' and Ashvaghosa speaks of songs sung to the acompment of the *mridanga* and of music produced on *mridangas* struck by the fingers of women, and the 'Lalitavistara' mentions it again and again with other varieties of drums.

I am inclined to think that Vatsyayana's *damaruka* stands here for percussion instruments in general. The *vina* even then formed the most popular of the musical instruments in India, as is apparent from the fact that it formed a necessary piece of furniture in the rooms of every Nagaraka on which, as we have seen, he played almost every evening. Such a *vina* in the room of Nanda reminds the bereaved Sundari of her dear absent husband, and Bhasa's Charudatta is overwhelmed by its merits and is enthusiastic in its praises.

Of wind instruments, the flute made of a bamboo reed (*vamsa*) is mentioned by Vatsyayana who praises it as capable of winning the heart of any girl when used in the way he prescribes. In the 'Buddhacharita' and 'Lalitavistara' it is called *venu* and is generally associated with the *vina* and women play upon it. We have seen that music with or without dances was enjoyed by our Nagaraka every evening. The Nagaraka's sons received lessons in music at the *gandharvashala* or college of music belonging perhaps to the city or to the *gana* or coporation to which he belonged. Sweet and ravishing songs delighting the ear, form, according to Vatsyayana, the readiest means of gaining the love of a man or a woman, and sometimes songs were specially composed containing a mention of the name and the family of the lover.

Concerts (*turyya*) are mentioned by Vatsyayana, in which a party of musicians of both sexes sang and played together on various instruments. A party of such players

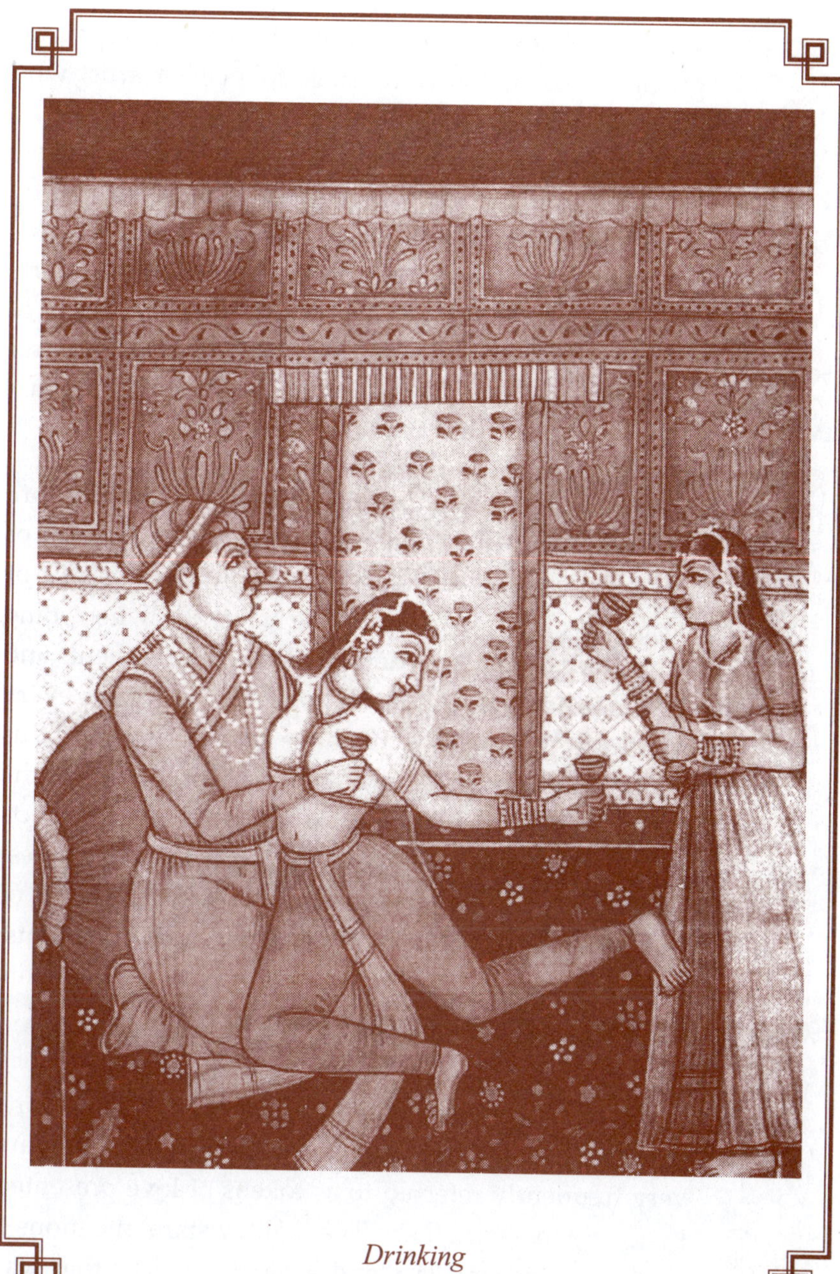

Drinking

was sometimes strengthened by its head (*rangopajivin*) giving his daughter in marriage to a clever artist who could help in the concert. An actress is mentioned by Vatsyayana as a very good carrier of love messages, because as Charudatta says, a person making a living by the *kalas*, like her, must be very clever at all sorts of tricks. Bharata says that sometimes on the stage the female parts were acted by men and an actress sometimes acted that of a man. Some actresses were maintained by the king and suitable quarters in the palace were set apart for them.

Crafts

In a society where both men and women wore ornaments, it was quite natural that the crafts of the jeweller (*manikara*) and goldsmith (*sauvarnika* or *suvarnakara*) should prosper. The Nagaraka, when going to his club or to his garden-picnic, wore ornaments and the king did so on his formal visit to the queens every afternoon. The statues that have come down from this age bear this out. It was, however, the demands of the ladies, who could not appear before their husbands without having ornaments on, that furnished the amplest occupation to the goldsmith and the jeweller. Some of theladies decorated their whole person with ornaments. Those who could not afford to have pure gold ornaments had to be satisfied with those made of an inferior kind of gold alloyed with an inferior metal.

Beyond a general mention of the *alamkaras* Vatsyayana does not name other ornaments than rings which are very frequently referred to as tokens of love presented by lovers to each other. The 'Lalitavistara' mentions a ring worth several lacs and a pearl necklace that was worth many times that sum. Charudatta's wife also had a pearl necklace given to her by her parents worth a lac. The testing of jewels and coin (*rupya-ratna-pariksa*) was a uselful art in this community and Vatsyayana knows a Vaikatika, a diamond-cutter, whose craft was to purify or refine precious stones. Plates and other vessels made of the precious metals, gold and silver, are mentioned by Vatsyayana and were evidently often used in the houses of the rich while those made of the baser metals, copper, bell-metal or iron, were used by ordinary people. Moreover, vessels made of earth, split-bamboo, wood and skins were in very general use.

Besides the jeweller, the goldsmith and the diamond cutter, the dyer of clothes *(ranjaka)* also was an artisan who appears to have access to the inner apartment of the Nagaraka's house and to take orders from the ladies direct. Blue and orange (colour of the Kusumbha flower) seem to be the dyes most fashionable; the dyer is by preference called the *nilikusumbha-ranjaka.* The yellow dye was also perhaps generally used, though the dye obtained from turmeric (*haridra*) provides a proverbial expression for denoting fickle, impermanent affection. Sundari, Nanda's beloved wife, is described as weaving a garment of the colour of the ruby (*padmaraga*) which is no doubt the same as the *kusukmbha* colour of Vatsyayana, and in the 'Buddhacharita' a lady is represented wearing a blue dress. Earlier still, these very same dyes appear to have been in favour. The noble Licchavi youths who went out of Vesali to pay their respects to the great Buddha are described in the 'Mahavagga' as wearing blue, red and yellow robes besides white ones; the same work enumerates a number of other colours being used by people living in the enjoyments of the world, though even

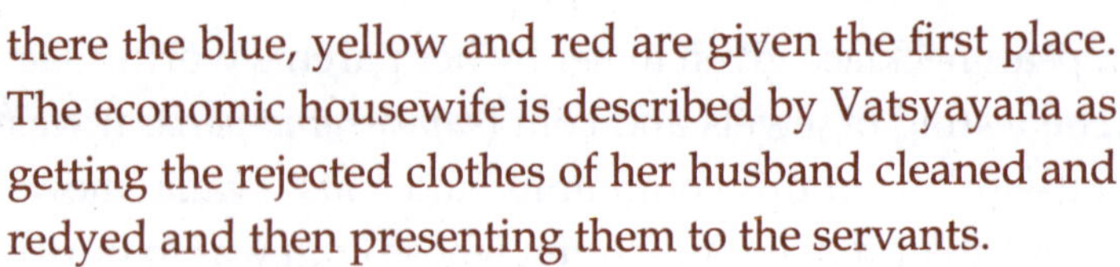

there the blue, yellow and red are given the first place. The economic housewife is described by Vatsyayana as getting the rejected clothes of her husband cleaned and redyed and then presenting them to the servants.

A number of artisans are mentioned by Vatsyayana as helping the Nagaraka in the decoration of his person and thus in his quest of love, and are spoken of by Vatsyayana as his friends: among them we find in the first place, the florist who looks after his flowerbeds, who makes garlands for his neck and chaplets for his head, and who helps him in preparing floral decorations for presentations to his beloved.

Next comes the perfumer *(saugandhika)* whom, as we have seen, he patronized very liberally. Then we have the goldsmith, the betelleaf-seller, as also the washerman, the barber and the wine-seller. The womenfolk of these artisans were also regarded by him as his friends (*mitram*). This establishment of friendly relations between the wealthy Nagaraka and the craftsmen appears to indicate a great respect for the crafts which are nowhere in Vatsyayana spoken of as implying any inferior rank or position.

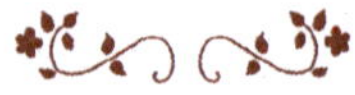